Recovery Is...

...journeys to wellbeing

A collection of individual interpretations on the meaning of Recovery

HUBB Mental Health User Group

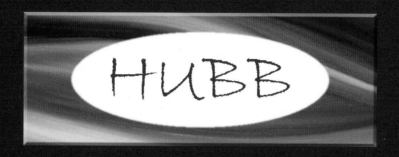

Published by HUBB Mental Health User Group

109 Rose Lane, Romford, Essex RM6 5NR United Kingdom

www.hubbmentalhealth.co.uk
T: +44 (0) 208 590 2666

First published 2011

ISBN: 978-09569603-0-6

Printed by Metloc Printers Limited. Romford, Essex

Contents

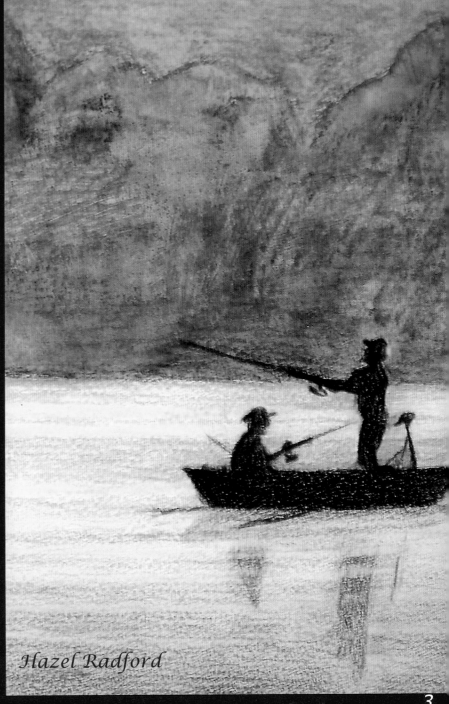

Hazel Radford

HUBB VALUES

Informed Choice For ALL!

Expert Knowledge

Support

True Consultation

Focus on Skills

Informative

Appropriate & Timely

RECOVERY FOCUSED

RECOVERY IS CENTRAL

ACTIVE LISTENING

VISION

PROMOTE INDEPENDENCE

MOVING PEOPLE FORWARD

Not The Label

Keep Other Services Grounded

Approachable

Value Everyone

Responsive

Non-Judgemental

Empowerment

Empathy

Foreword to 'Recovery Is...'

The 'Recovery Is' book is a celebration of much of the work undertaken by HUBB and those who support our work on our 20th Anniversary as a service user-led organisation. HUBB began in August 1991 as people were being discharged into the community from the old mental health asylums. It was felt that going into 'new territory', a community organisation would be needed to help with the transition to support people in their new lives.

The recovery theme came from the mental health service user movement and has now become mainstream policy. This book hopefully demonstrates the pure essence of recovery which is often misunderstood by those who think they can convert the recovery approach to a 'model'.

This book celebrates the 'ordinary' things that people do to stay well on their recovery journey. When people become mentally unwell, they never lose their skills; they lose their self belief and their confidence. The content of this book is designed to show how people have regained both. Recovery is often misunderstood and misinterpreted by many. It is self-defining and unique to the person.

Most people's recovery journeys are not straightforward, but I hope you will see that by doing the 'ordinary' the contributors have been transformed into 'extraordinary' people, with the power to inspire others to take the first tentative steps on their own recovery path.

> *"When at some point in our lives, we meet a real tragedy, we can react in one of two ways. Obviously, we can lose hope and let ourselves slip into despair, into alcohol, drugs, or unending sadness. Or else we can wake ourselves up, discover in ourselves an energy that was hidden there, and act with greater clarity and more force.*
>
> *Anyone who feels overwhelmed has no power over reality. Knowing how to accept the blows dealt by fate means never giving up"*
>
> *His Holiness the Dalai Lama (2002) 'The Spirit of Peace'*

This book will be distributed widely to help inspire others to discover their hidden energies.

The fact that HUBB has existed for twenty years is a testament to the Committee, staff, and most of all the people who use our services, who have 'never given up' trying to improve mental health services, and their own experiences of managing distress.

Jenny Gray - HUBB Director

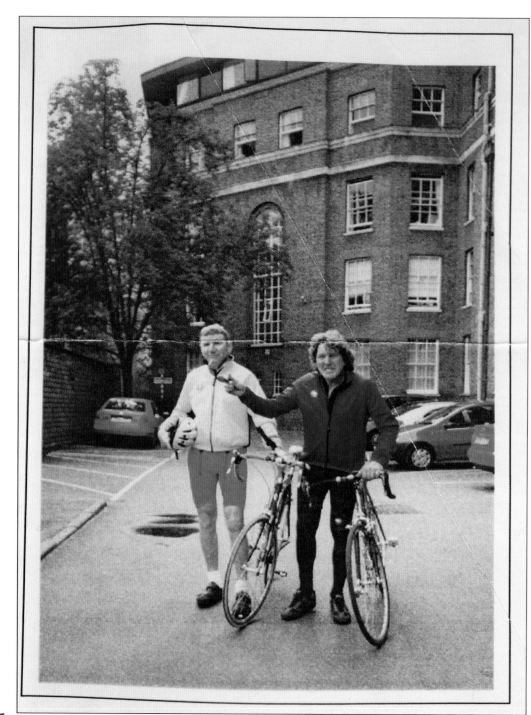

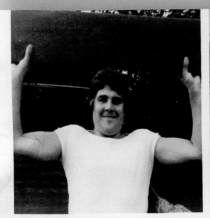

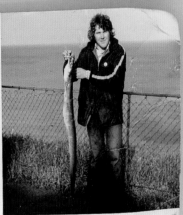

Praise my soul the King of heaven

Praise, my soul, the King of heaven,
To his feet thy tribute bring;
Ransomed, healed, restored, forgiven,
Who like me his praise should sing?
Alleluia! Alleluia!
Praise the everlasting King.

Praise him for his grace and favour
To our fathers in distress;
Praise him still the same as ever,
Slow to chide, and swift to bless:
Alleluia! Alleluia!
Glorious in his faithfulness.

Father-like, he tends and spares us,
Well our feeble frame he knows;
In his hands he gently bears us,
Rescues us from all our foes:
Alleluia! Alleluia!
Widely as his mercy flows.

Angels, help us to adore him;
Ye behold him face to face;
Sun and moon, bow down before him,
Dwellers all in time and space:
Alleluia! Alleluia!
Praise with us the God of grace.

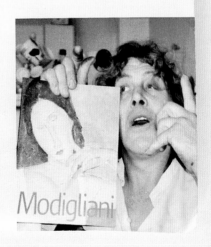

This book is dedicated to the memory of Robert Michael Charles Harrison.

He described himself as:

- A Poet
- An Artist
- A Carpenter
- An Ordinary Man

Donations in Robert's memory enabled HUBB to purchase a number of digital cameras which helped some members create contributions for this project.

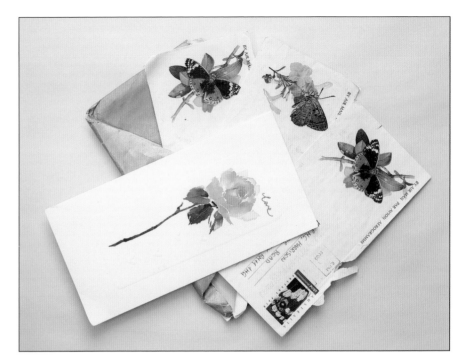

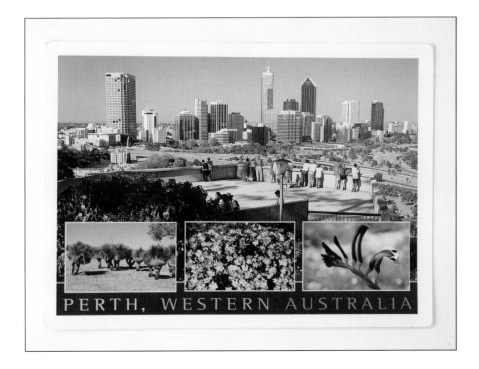

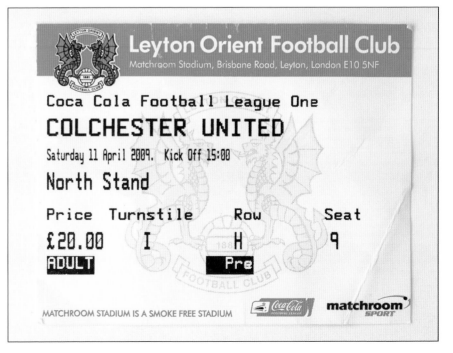

Recovery Is...

Seeing The Positive

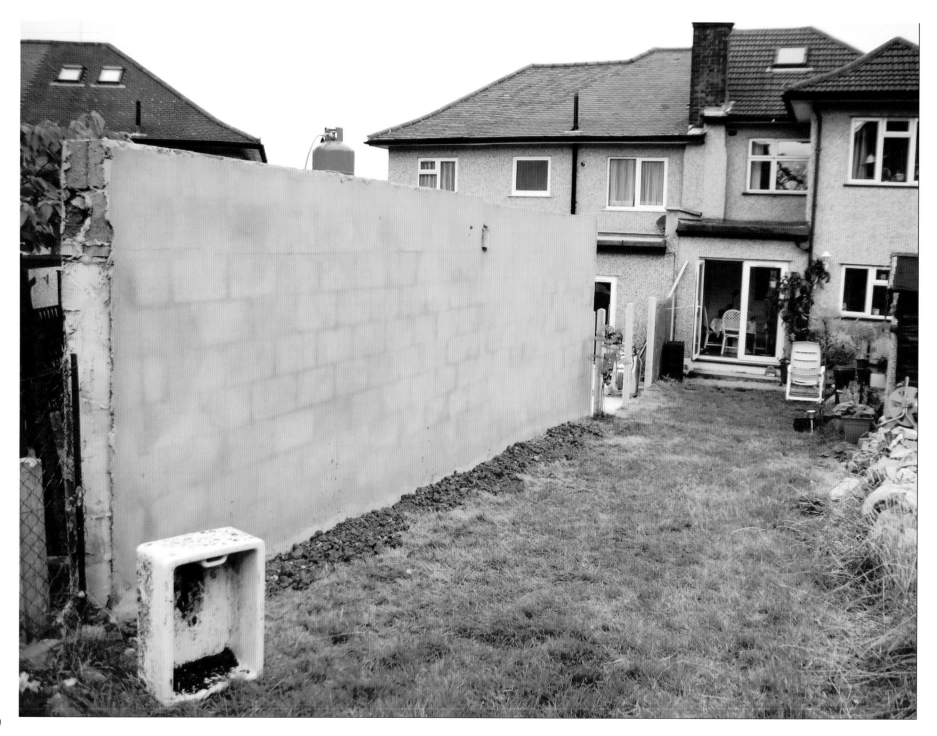

My neighbours moved to Essex from the East End of London to enjoy the 'country'.

They built this wall.

The wall, to me, is a sign of London expanding. Concrete, city, business first!

Nature second!

Other people have been annoyed because they once looked out and saw green. Now they see a wall.

I was asked what I thought of this. When I really thought...I could see a blank canvas staring at me!

Neighbour against neighbour.
I alone can't save the planet
I'll be creative! I have a plan!
I'll soften the view with plants.
A garden design with bamboo
A trellis
An old window frame
A window box to grow strawberries or herbs
A bench to sit on
A pergola as a garden feature
Plenty of plant pots too!

I'm getting excited!
I know what to do!

I refuse to see this wall as negative!!!

Denise Miller

The Wall

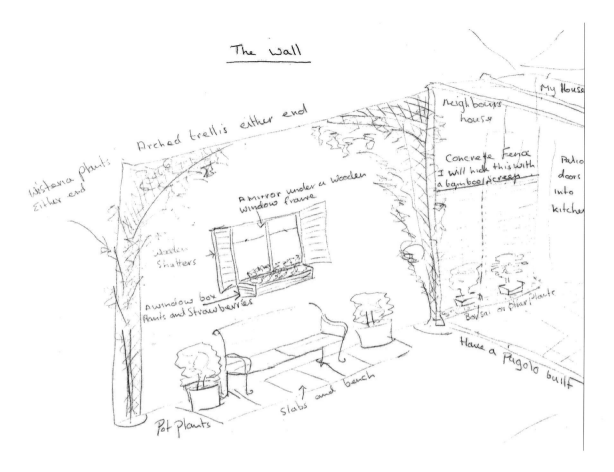

Arched trellis either end

Wisteria plants Either end

A mirror under a wooden window frame

Wooden Shutters

A window box Plants and Strawberries

Neighbours house

Concrete Fence I will hide this with a bamboo screen

My House

Patio doors into kitchen

Bonsai or other plants

Have a Pugolo built

Pot plants

Slabs and bench

I refuse to see this wall as a negative that divids people. Here is my solution and how I will make this wall a symbol of togetherness and a positive outlook.

I love the potential of a drab concrete wall offering the creativity to producing an oasis of calm. A bright future.

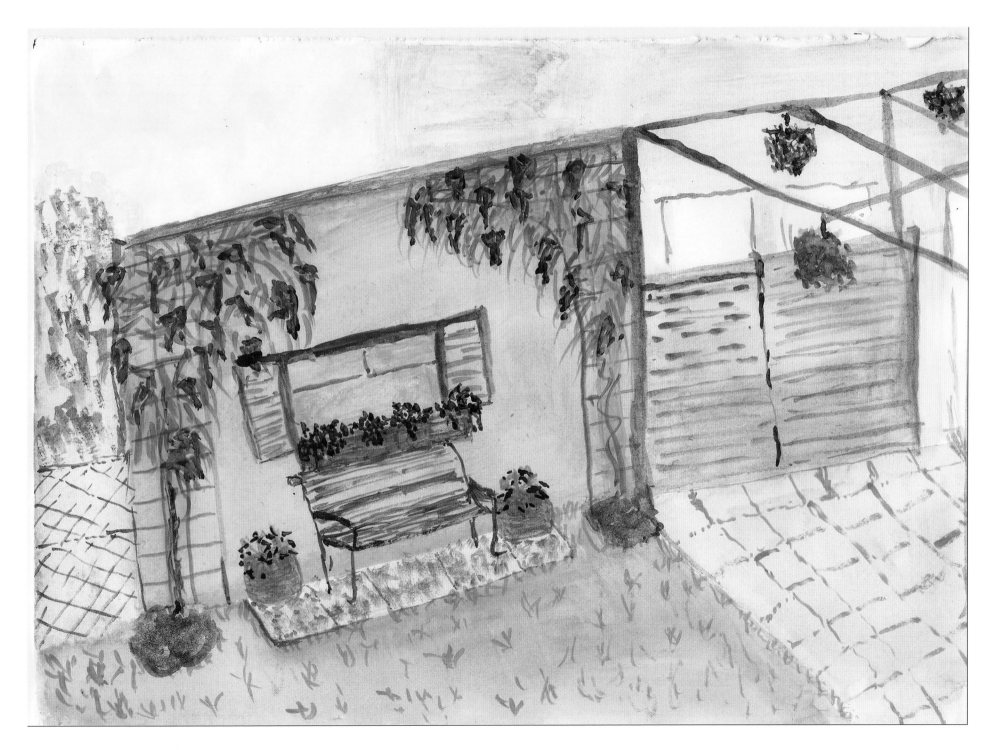

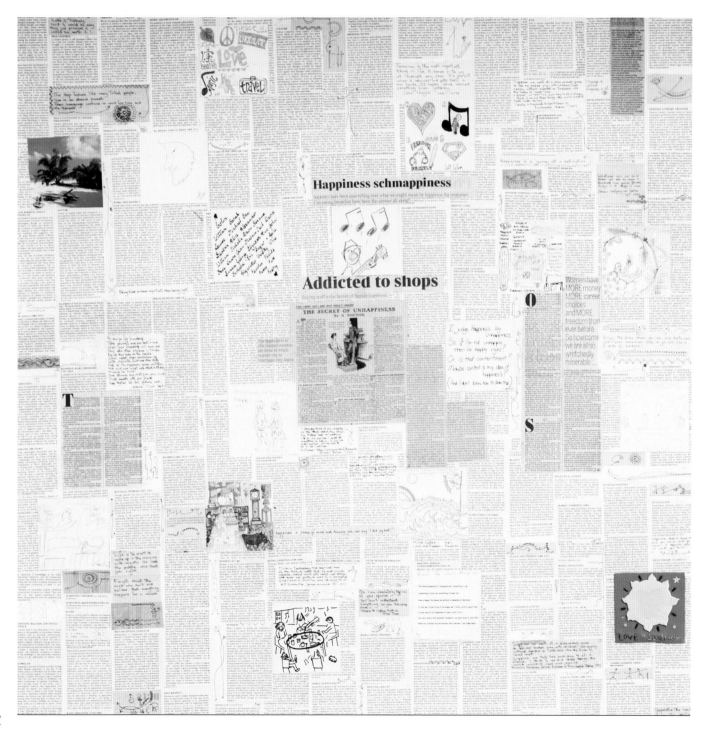

Lyn Jones

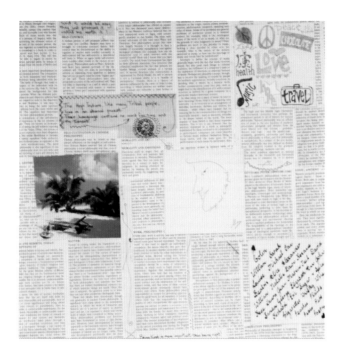

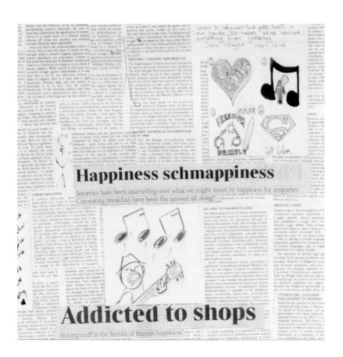

Happiness schmappiness

Addicted to shops

Your space...your happiness square.
Fill it with what makes you happy!

Recovery Is...

Poetry

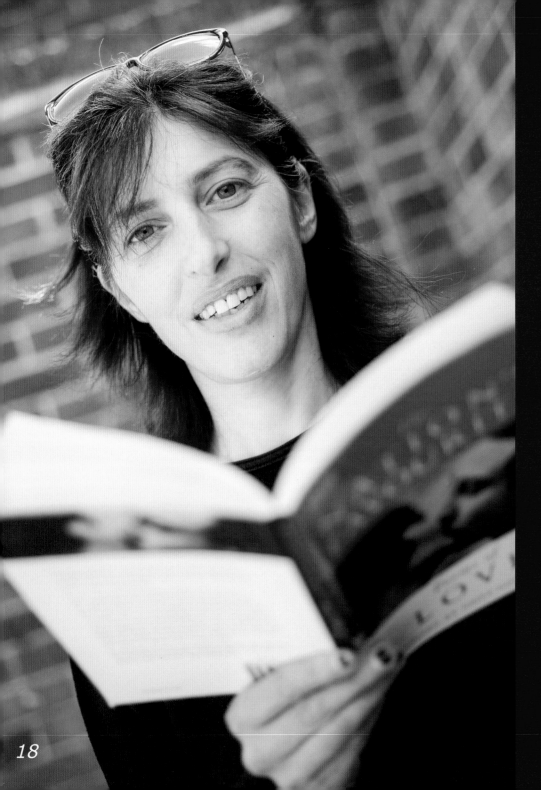

'When I read poetry...

I feel I'm in another world...

A different world'

'Here I am reading one of my favourite poems:

Sonnet from the Portuguese XLIII
Elizabeth Barratt Browning (1806 - 1862)'

Gisella Patrizia Elena Agosti

You

You are what you think you are
so watch your thoughts each day.

Believe completely in yourself
and don't be led astray

By the things that other people say and do
always remember this: unto yourself be true.

There is a law that operates
behind the passing show

Every little thing you do
you reap exactly what you sow.

So if you don't believe in everthing you do
how can you expect others to believe and value you?

Anonymous

Dark & Light

A blind's pulled down to separate
Outside is love inside is hate
Hate is dark but love is light
To raise the blind would be too bright
But gradually small holes appear
And beams of light dispel the fear
The dark's not black it's only grey
And getting lighter by the day
The holes expand the blind gets thin
More love and light come pouring in
One day the blind will fall apart

And light and love will fill my heart

Susan Spelling

Thought

Thinking and thinking and thinking again
Out of control like a runaway train
Gathering Speed and momentum and force
You tell me to stop but I just can't of course
Stuck on the rails and thundering on
Into the distance where all hope is gone
Too fast to get off I stay to the end
Past where my thoughts go right round the bend
A crash and a smash and I'm broken once more
Bloodied and bruised and battered and sore
My body is whole but my mind's in a mess
A familiar place of pain and distress

But I'm not alone cos you're waiting for me
When I lift up my eyes it's you that I see
I believe you can help and I trust in your word
I'll cling to the promise you gave and I heard
Help me break up these rails so my thinking is free
To find who I am so I can be me

Susan Spelling

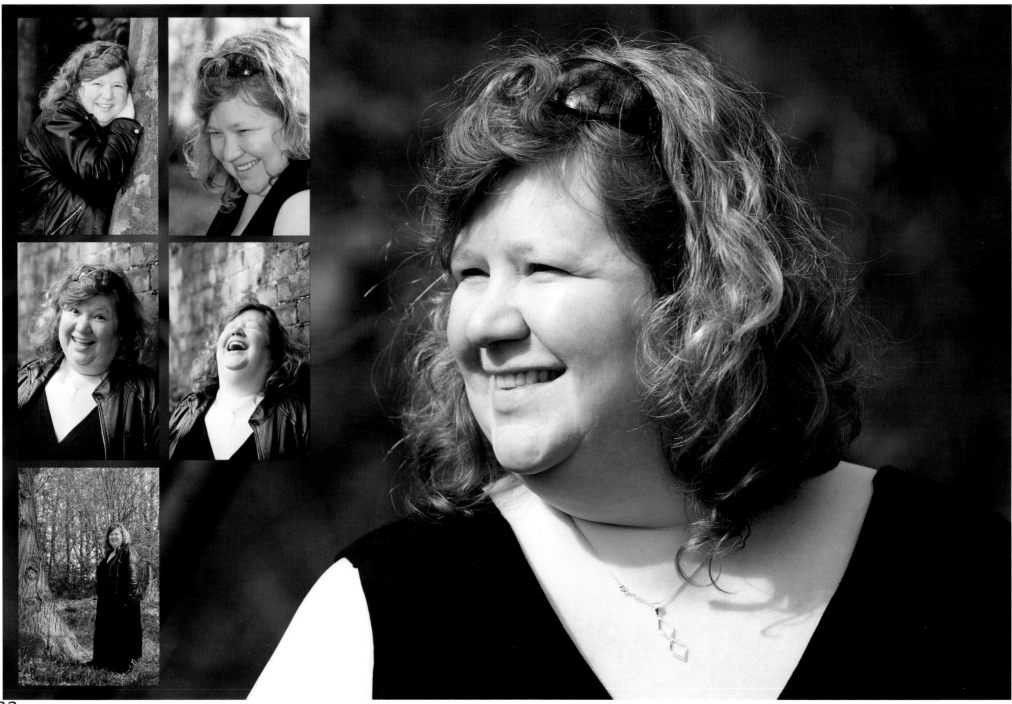

The Demon and Recovery....

This demon came and joined me on a very sunny day.

Where the demon came from
No one would dare say!

The demon came with many
turning my life desolate and grey.
One demon said: end your life if you want us to go away.

Mum came with armour telling those demons to go!
But the demons were having none of it; they were here to stay!

I was taken to a dungeon where more demons would say
take this medication if want them to go away.

I was looking out of a dark window where I saw a light.
I thought if I'm going to face those demons I'm going to have to fight.

I met a woman from a user group with the same bright light.
Take the number of this woman she will help you with your fight!

I met with this woman on that same strange day; who said
I believe in your demons but they have been with you before that sunny day.

These demons who had joined me were indeed my friends,
who had come to say if you do not face them they will never go away!

These demons I now know were feelings deep inside.
Learning to embrace them and never, never hide.

Then when those demons visit me on a bright and sunny day.
I now know how to deal with them and send them on their way.

Lynn Burling

Chocolat

Chocola-chocola
Crumbling onto my moist tongue
Flaky, dulling my pain
Devoured by me first in the Belgium Congo
Belgium truffles enticing, my wet mouth
Scooping the aura of smooth cream vanilla
Oozing honey-sweet caramel
Dark coal, white snow within hard centres
And baby-soft edges
Sparkling diamonds in diamante boxes
Chocola-chocola
Beckoning me in the deep, dark, silent night
Comforting me in the crystal, clear, daylight
Cholola-Chocola
Rolling round and round my tongue
A secret hidden at the bottom of my drawer
Chocola-chocola
You are the love that betrays my thighs
And brings tear-drops to my wide eyes
Chocola-chocola
My Valentine

Fatima Kassam

hubb

hubb are like a life line
they're dagenham now not mine
but when they worked with me in havering
they made my mental health shine

if it wasn't for dinah from hubb
the dispute with the electric would never end
if it wasn't for my advocates
society would have driven me round the bend

although funding for havering has ended
i have now learnt how to cope
and knowing if i go into hospital
they'll still help me and i'll have hope

we still meet up every month
for a buffet, raffle and talk
we meet up in romford baptist church
from the bus stop it's a short walk

every month we have a different topic
and staff that turn up each time
good old hubb i'll always say
and that's the end of my rhyme

Anonymous HUBB service user

A Prayer

To Strive, for a way out that brings
about sanity, serenity and peace

To Seek, a light that will burn so bright
it will cast away all darkness and shadows

To Find, instead of despair forever grinding away
at any thoughts of optimism or hope

And not to Yield, to voices that urge harm
but to fight back by blocking them out

To Recover, by finding the light that is sought
leading to the way out that is striven for

Robin Dixon

Soap-Opera-Drama

Soap-Opera-Drama
Called life
World won't change
Change yourself
Soap-Opera-Drama
My man's a cheating
My kids are hungry
The debt collectors knocking
Soap-Opera-Drama
War on T.V.
Earthquakes killing kids in Haiti
Parents injured in Chile
The Final Age of Holy Books
Soothsayer's predictions
Nostradamus's Visions
Age of hate, greed and envy
Kill or be killed
Don't mess with me
Soap-Opera-Drama
See my bling
Don't it shine?
It ain't mine
Soap-Opera-Drama
I want to die
But dying isn't easy
Soap-Opera-Drama
My mother loved me
Soap-Opera-Drama
Called Life

Fatima Kassam

Recovery Is...

About People

Recovery Is…Having Friends

Friends can be an invaluable source of mental wellbeing. But quality rather than quantity must be the yardstick; better to have one good, honest friend than a whole battalion of fair-weather ones.

Since becoming a carer, my social contacts have diminished considerably, to the point of non-existence. However, as several doors have closed, one has opened where I have discovered a whole new set of friends. In truth, they are not new, having been around right under my nose all the time. It's simply that I have not appreciated them fully until recently. But, friends they are, undoubtedly.

I see them regularly at the Drop-in where I attend. It's called My Garden, and it represents a health centre and a social centre all in one, a place of activity and stimulation for both body and mind.

My friends there are numerous and varied: The robins, tits and finches that feed from the many seed containers dotted around; the bees and butterflies that dart and flit among the buddleia seeking its nectar; the water insects hovering over the pond; including the delicate dragonflies, glinting brightly in the warm sunshine; squirrels collecting for their winter larder; hedgehogs, voles and other small mammals who drop in from time to time; and the annual pilgrimage of the frogs, come to do their duty in perpetuating their species. The resident fish don't mind – there is room enough for all!

All are welcome. Spring, summer, autumn and winter sees many comings and goings, time to say goodbye to some friends, and be reacquainted with others. As the brilliant blooms and verdant trees make way for vivid, deep hues, fogs and bareness, it heralds the arrival of two special friends – leaves and snow. I have great fun with them. There is something deeply satisfying about the rustling, whooshing and crunching sounds that they make as I walk through freshly fallen carpets of both. They always lift my spirits.

Then there are the noisy extroverts who drop in unexpectedly with their bluster and energy. Enter thunder and lightning, galeforce winds and torrential rain. Yes, they can be a bit boisterous and over the top but they are still characters and it takes all sorts. Variety is the spice of life, they say!

Lastly, I have my intellectual friends, books, music and pencil, constant companions at my patio desk. The latter helps me record my thoughts and write my stories but all have an important input and are non-judgemental. I consider myself fortunate indeed to be surrounded by such an eclectic mix. And, in my case, the fair weather ones are as genuine as the inclement weather ones!

L.S.

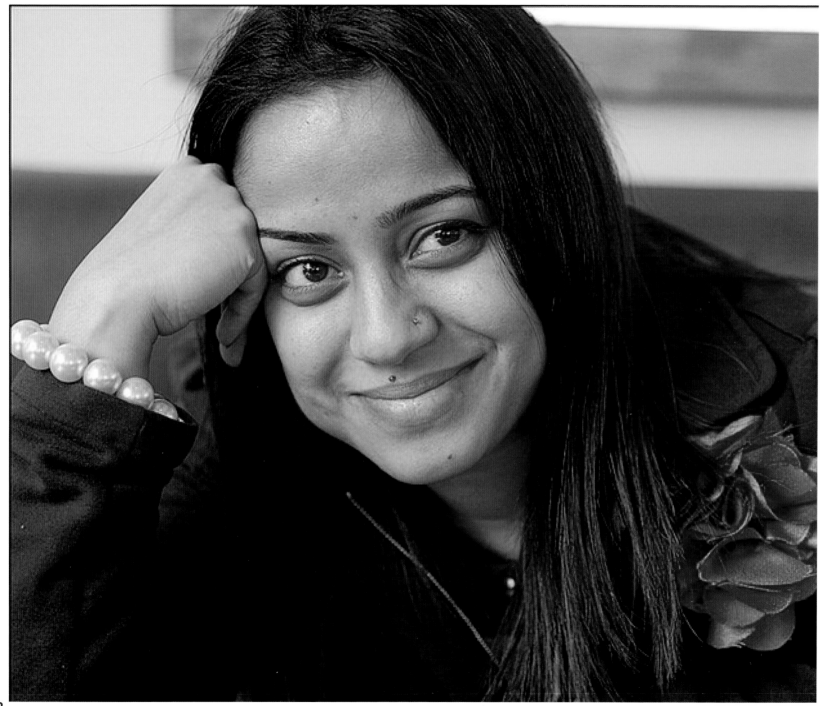

Recovery Is...

I keep well by sensing the environment around me, by being reminded explicitly and implicitly that I am thought about by the people I love. I keep positively motivated most by watching my children play. I love the joy me giving something to people around me has.

The images that depict this most closely are attached:

Message in jam
Message in sand
My children at play
My henna art proudly and symbolically displayed by my friend and girls.

Poppy Jaman

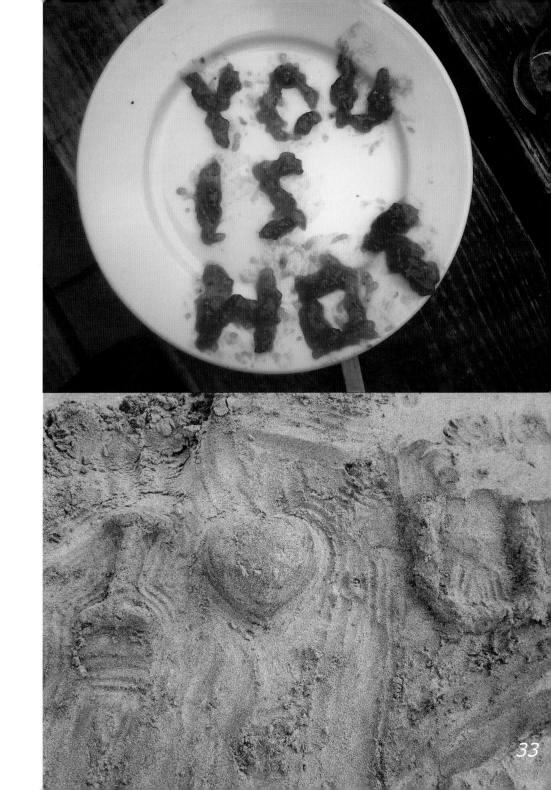

33

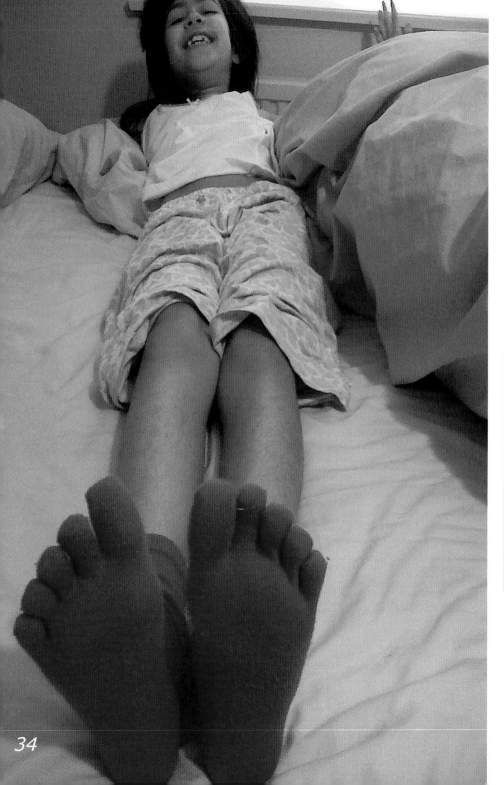
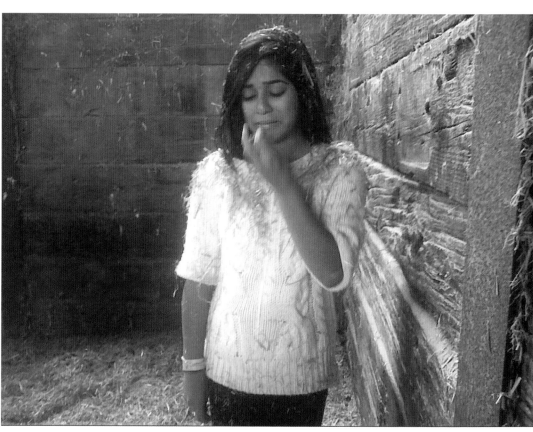

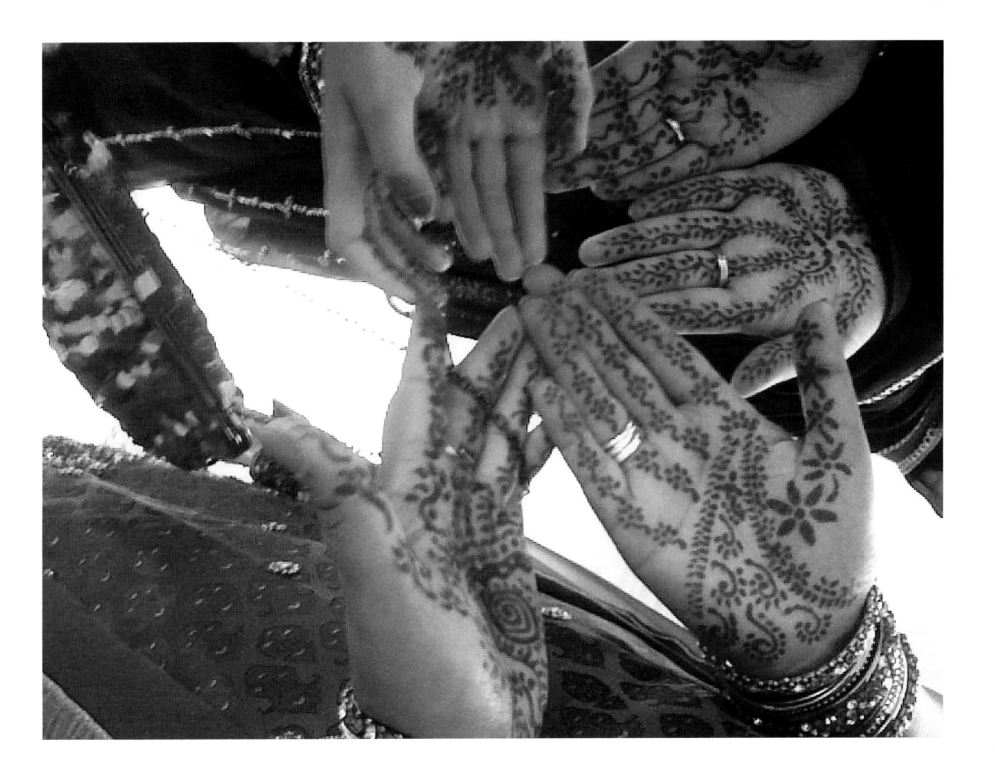

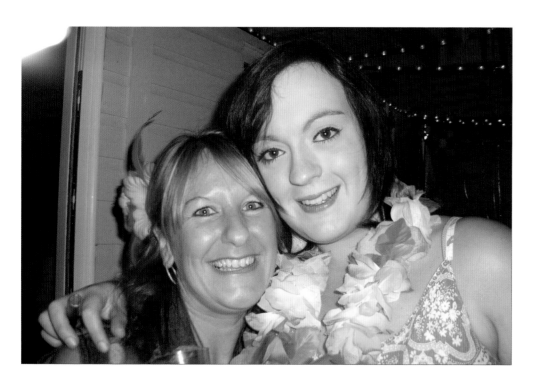

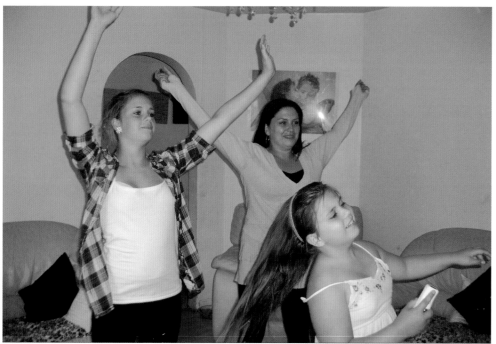

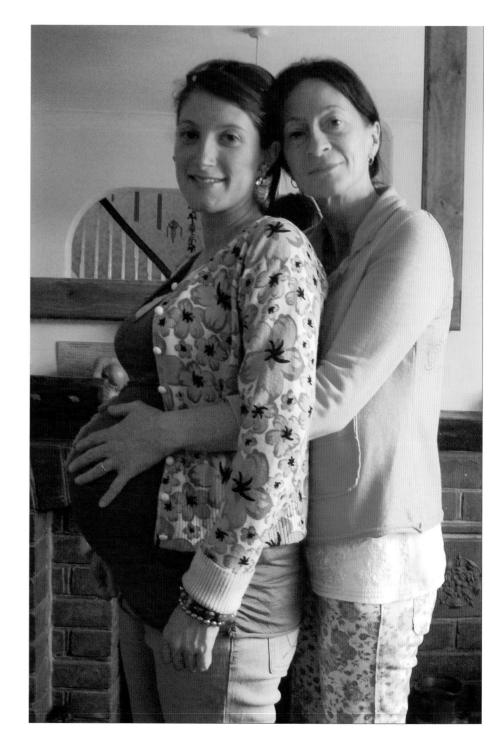

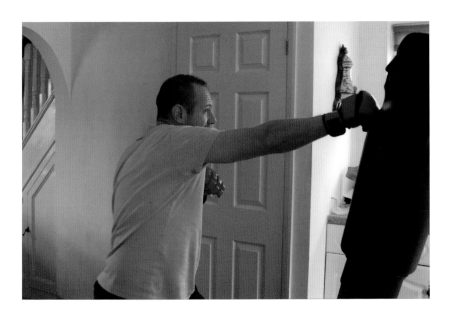

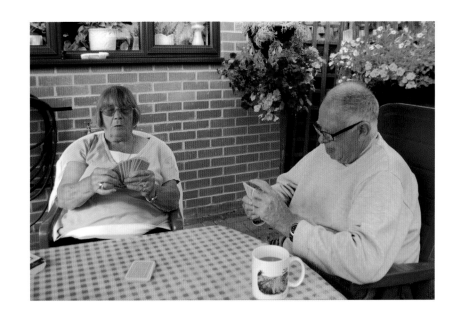

People In My Life

Denise Miller

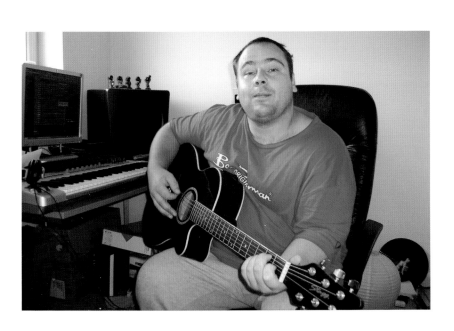

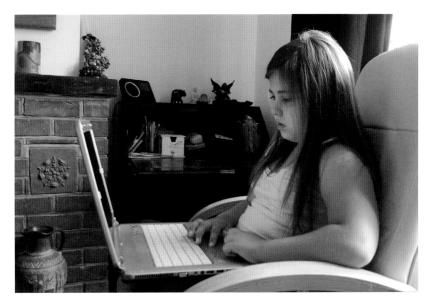

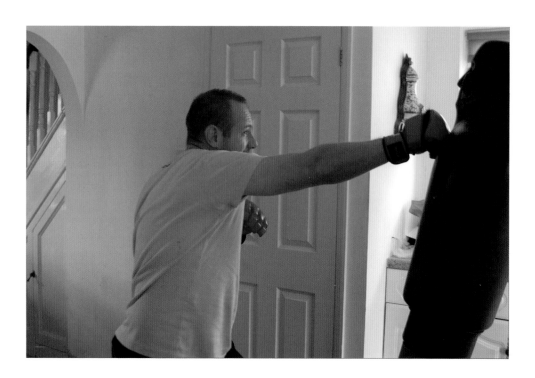

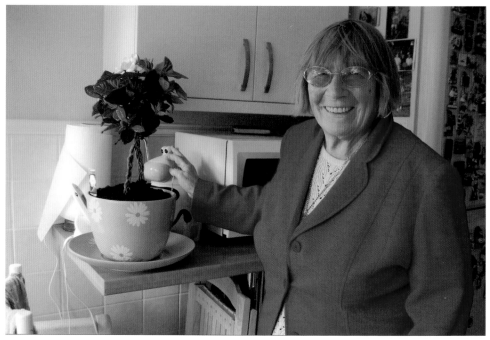

This is my son celine he likes keeping fit and has a lot of energy. He is a Guard in the White Tower of London. I am very Proud of him Love him to bits, he has a Great Sense of humour.

On mother's day my Sister and I bought a very large cup and Saucer that can be used as a Plant pot. This is our mum myra, She is Loved dearly. She is a Very kind Warm Lady.

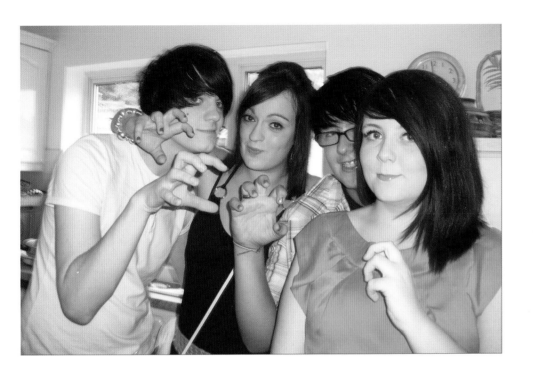

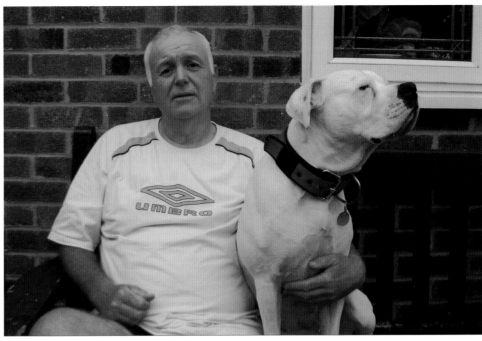

my daughter Sinead with
her friends Danny, Jon and
Georgia. Ready for Tuesday night
Clubing. They make me Laugh
Seeing their Sense of fun. I love
her, I'm her mum.

Friends remind me of my youth a Sense
of belonging, Nostalga my roots
Steve and Lily. a man and his dog
They are members of ACES Athletic
Canine Enthusiast Society. Lily races, aframe,
Long Jump and weight pulling Lure racing.
We have been friends with Steve and his
wife Terry since forever.

Recovery Is...

Art

Loving touch

Safety

A complete absence of fear and threat

Submerge myself in warmth

Being touched when like this is bliss

Rare

Wonder

Bliss

From 'Eight foundation stones of this gangrel recovery'
Jeremy Voaden

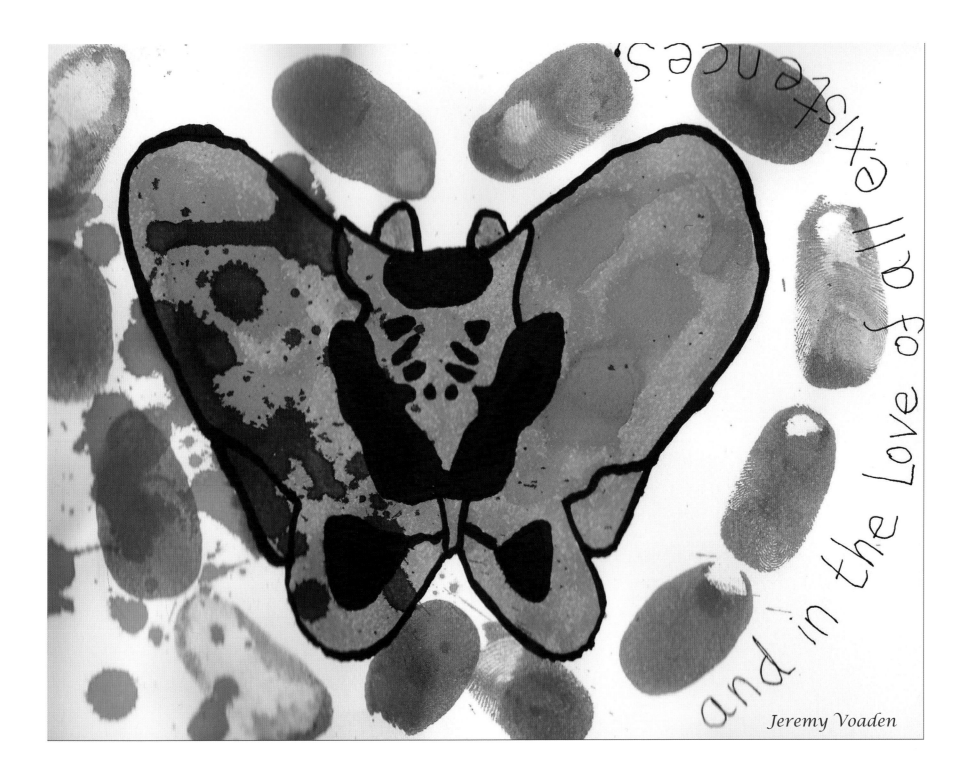

and in the Love of all existences.

Jeremy Voaden

43

I started painting as part of my recovery programme from severe depression and anxiety, quickly finding that I enjoyed it, benefiting in several ways.

It helped my concentration, as well as encouraging me to see detail in my surroundings and I soon began to see a natural beauty that lifted my spirits. The more my skills developed, through help from a patient art teacher, the more my confidence grew and I began to try differing artistic mediums.

Now I have returned part time to the work place and college, painting gives me valuable relaxation time vital to me maintaining my well being. I have recently successfully applied for a place on the degree programme in mental health nursing which I will start in March 2012.

When I qualify I hope I can use art as a positive way of connecting with people I am supporting.

Julie Sheen

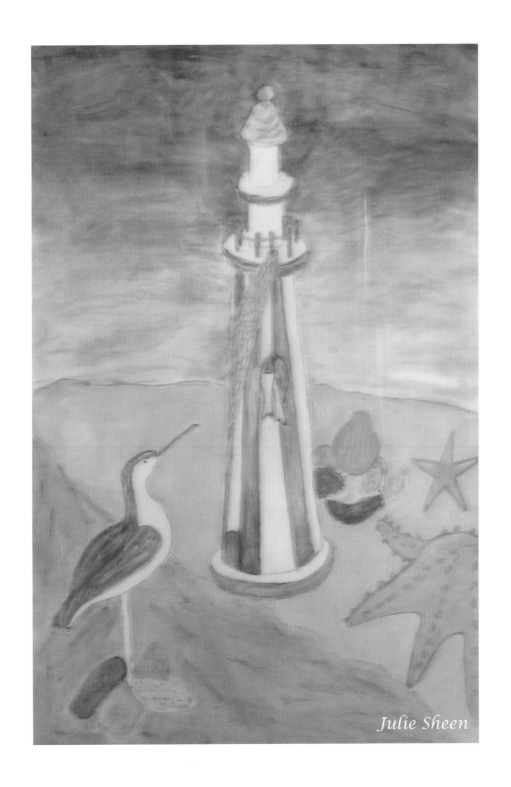

Julie Sheen

45

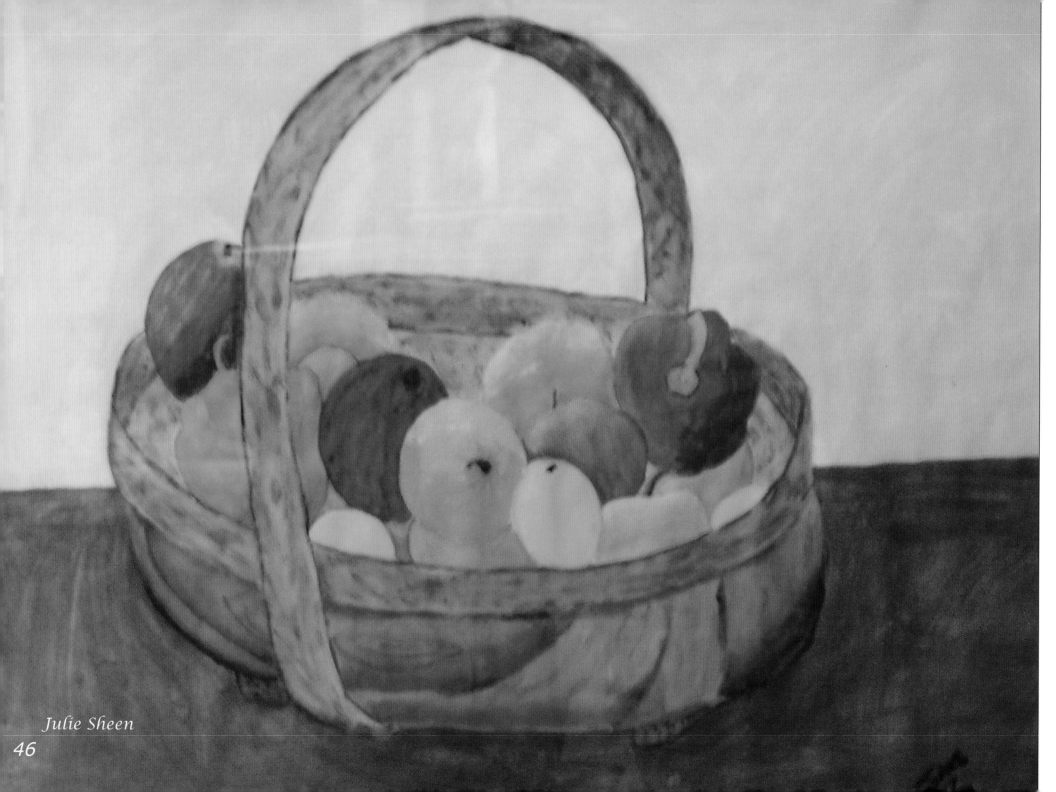

Julie Sheen

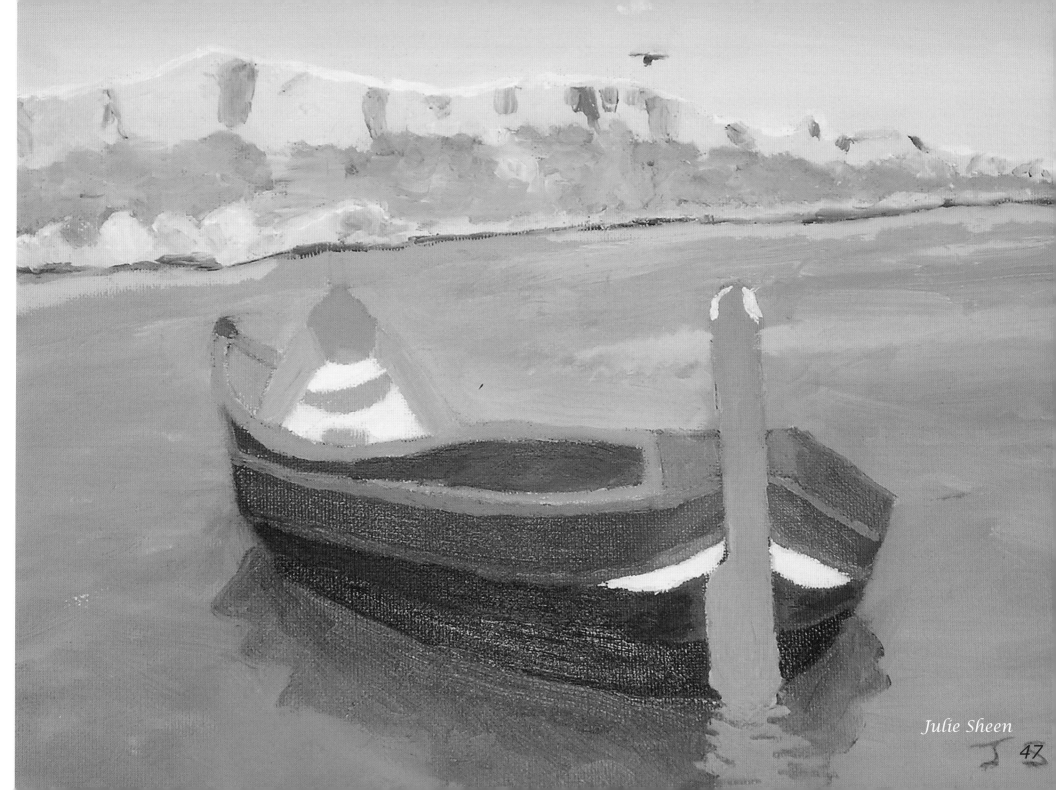

Julie Sheen

47

Recovery to me is reconciliation of loss.

Recovery is accepting things as they are.

Lyn Jones

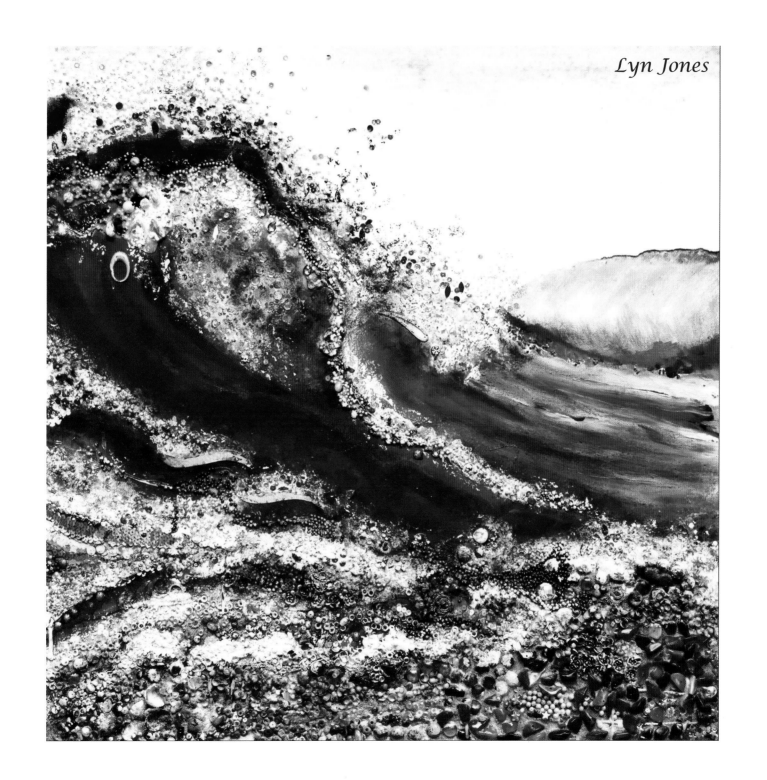

Lyn Jones

Happiness does not depend on who you are or what you have.

It depends solely on what you think.

For me Recovery was finding my independence.

Lyn Jones

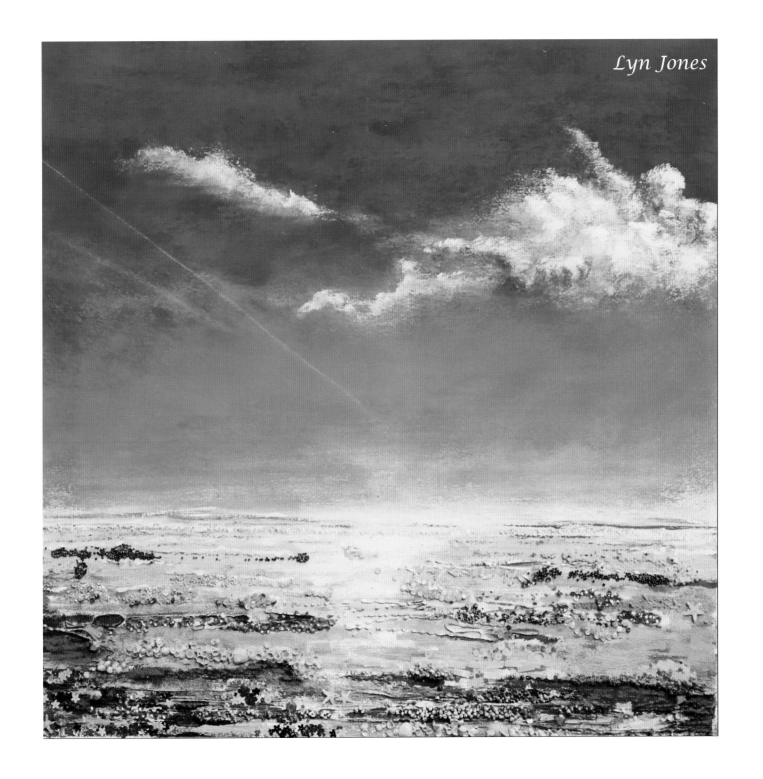

Lyn Jones

Independence of thought and the discovery that I like myself.

Being Happy in your own skin is the secret to living on your own.

Lyn Jones

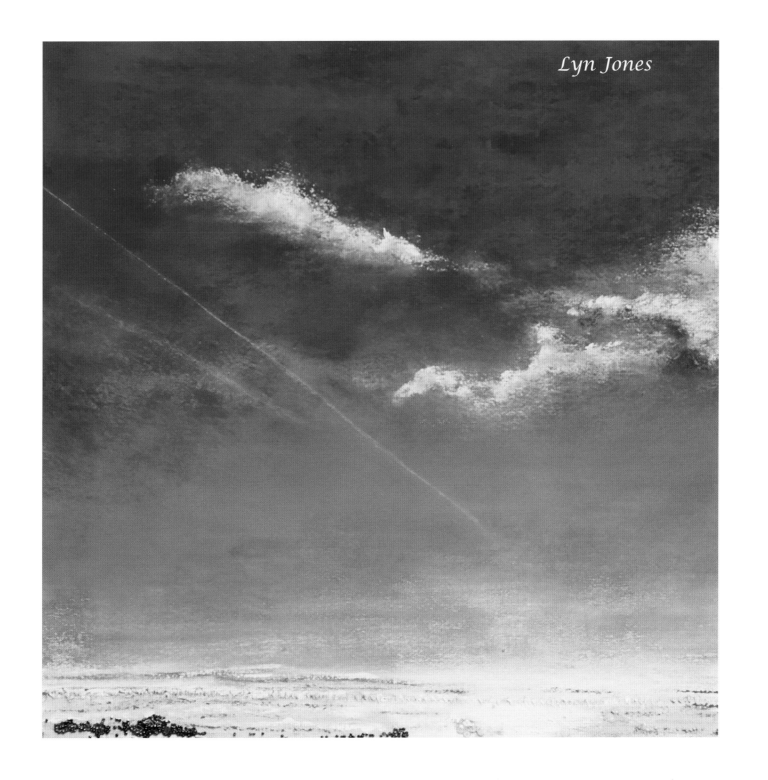

Lyn Jones

53

The Pictures Feed Me

A child takes a crayon or some paint and sets to the paper. No fear of judgement. I take my crayons and paints all about, bothies, hostels, megaliths, Premier Travel Inns. Frequently offer to share them if folk look interested. Often the response is "No thanks, I can't draw".

Everyone can draw, everyone can paint. Just putting the colours or lines down evidences this.

Making pictures is one of the few parts of my life where I do not feel subject to judgement myself or more accurately, judge myself hard.

It feels good to create mess, splash strong colour (purple is my favourite) and build thick layers of pigment on paper.

Look into the wonderful glutinous mix.

I don't care really what other people think about the pictures I make.

From 'Eight foundation stones of this gangrel recovery'
by Jeremy Voaden

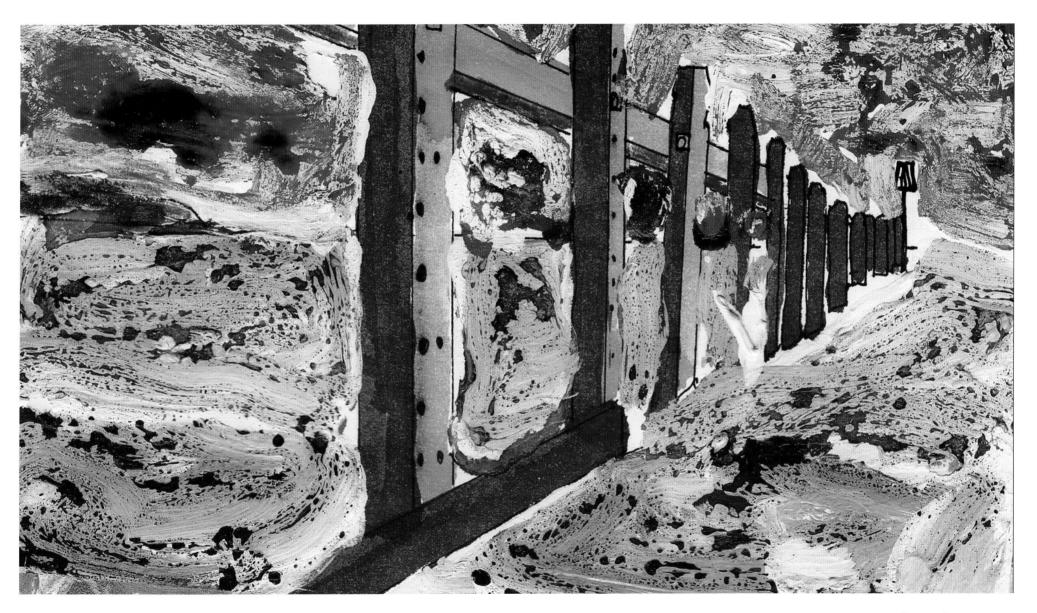

Jeremy Voaden

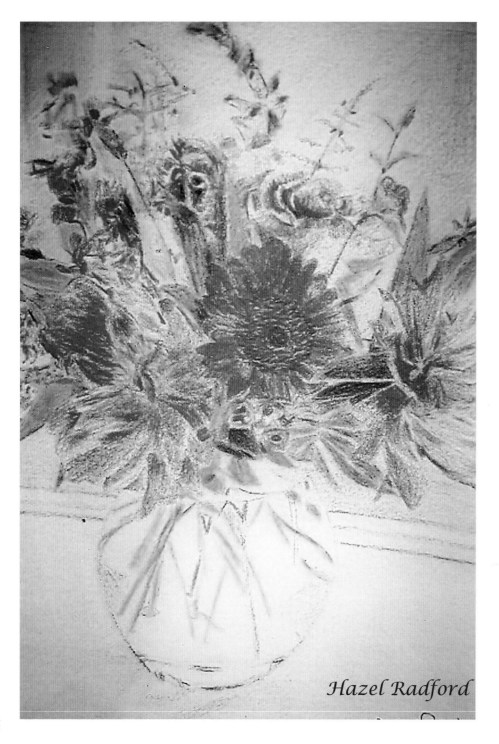

Hazel Radford

① The Fishing Trip
② Pretty Pink Flowers

I Enjoy artwork. This is because it is relaxing, creative and a pleasure for others to see the end product. It has helped keep me well, in times when I feel stressed. My artwork has helped me a great deal, with living with my mental health problems. My artwork has helped me in my recovery and possibly I have inspired others.

H J Radford
HAZEL RADFORD
H. J. RADFORD (MRS)

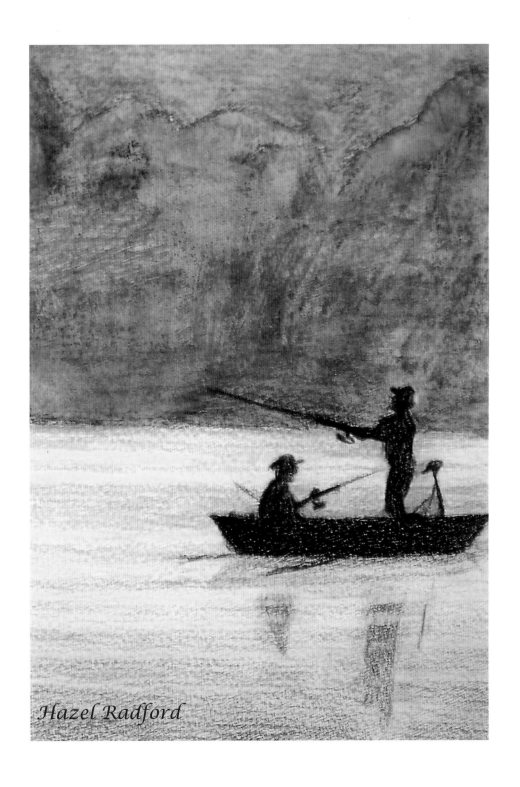

Hazel Radford

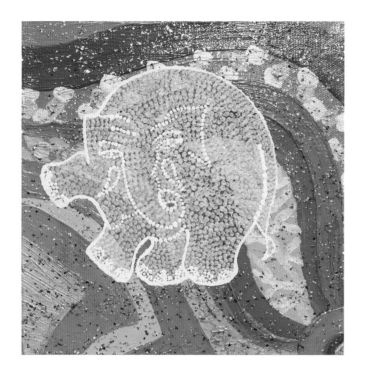
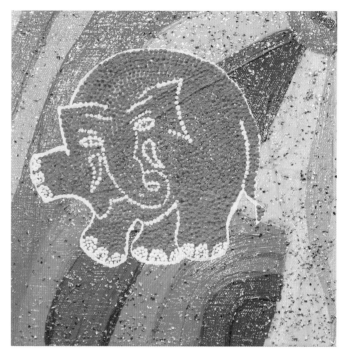
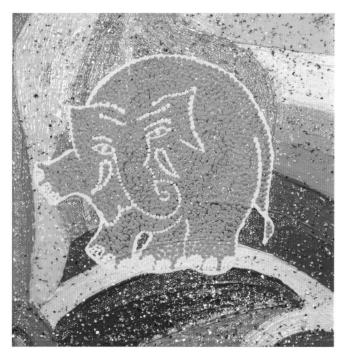
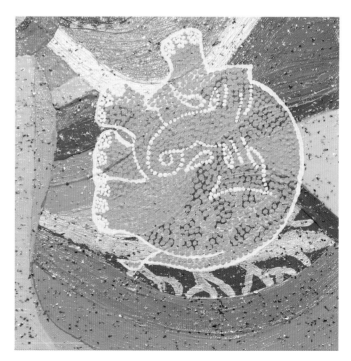

Katie Francis

58

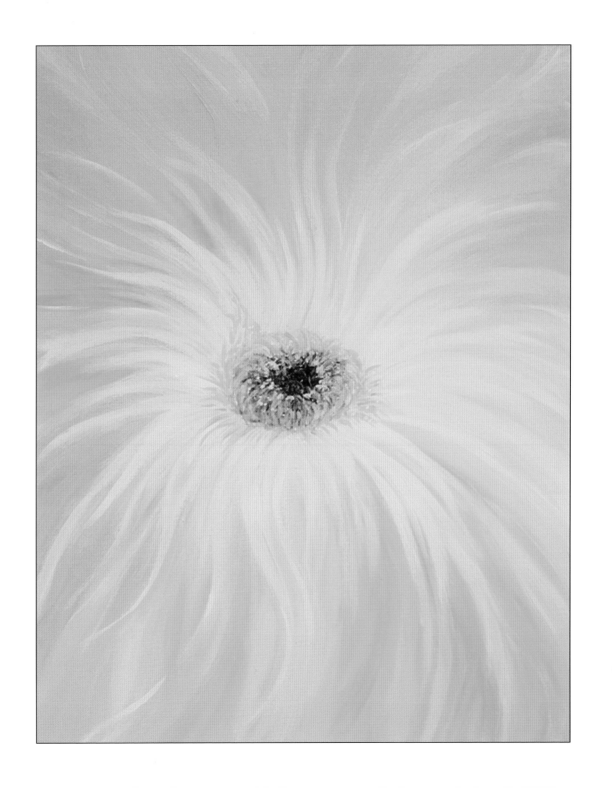

Michelle Griffiths
'Studio 3 Arts'

Recovery Is...

Thoughts

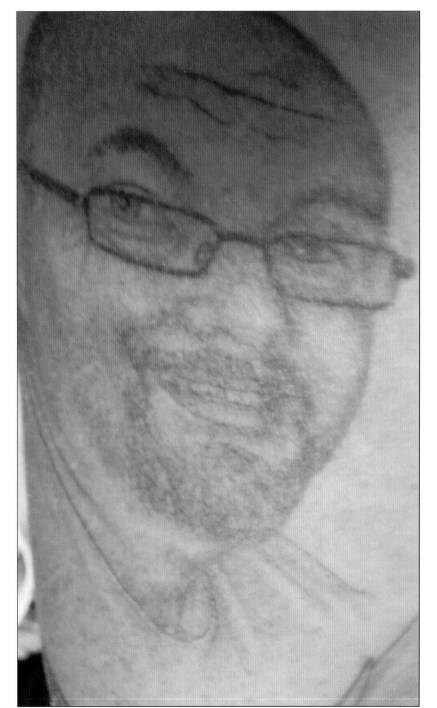

All Things Important

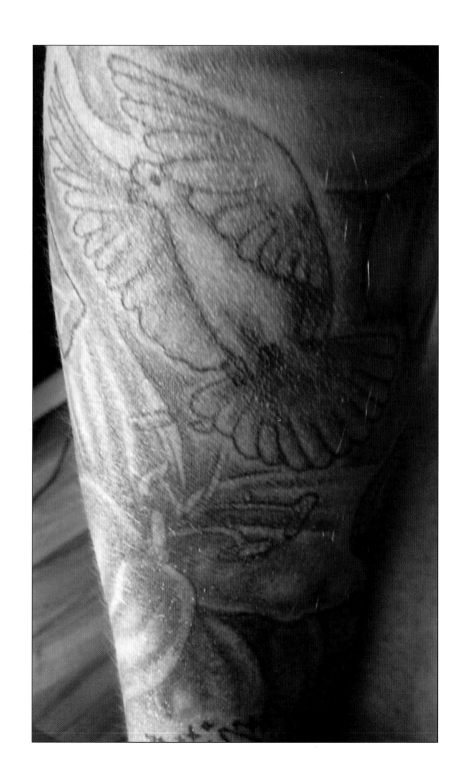

8 Years ago my life changed when I had to leave work and was diagnosed with Bipolar Disorder. The following years have been hard work but have been full of many rewards. I decided a few years ago to have all the things that are important in my life, tattoo'd on my arm in a sleeve. I carry with me at all times these things that keep me strong and keep me well. Among them are my husband David, my son Davey, St. Dymphna the patron saint of mental illness. Also important to me is peace in my life so the doves represent that. My faith helps to keep me strong so I have the cross as well as lilies included. Everyday no matter where I am I am reminded of these wonderful things that have entered into my life during my bipolar journey and how they will always be there to keep me going. I love it when people ask about my tattoo…it gives me the chance to share my story with others. Strangers rarely stay strangers through my story.

Julie Drake

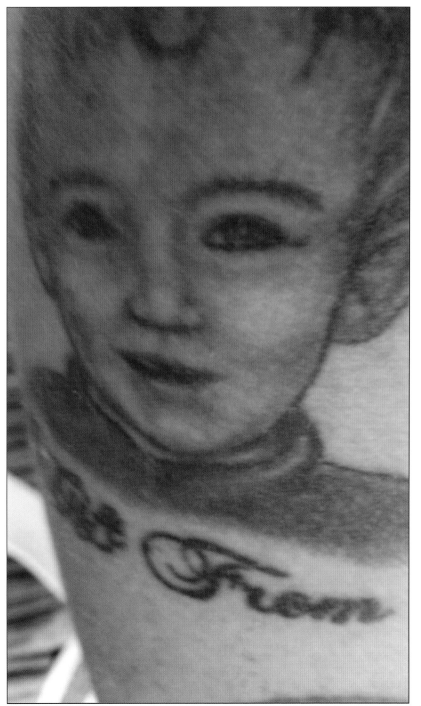

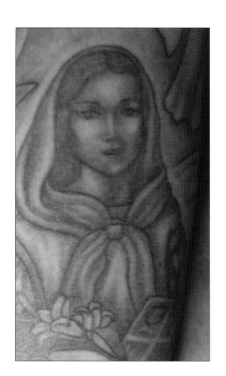

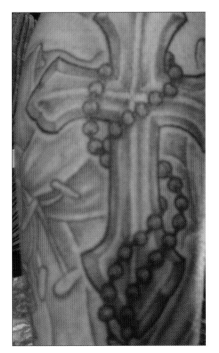

From the Struggle to 'Recovery'

When everyday is a struggle, you are trying your best to fight it, but it feels that you are stuck in an emotional quicksand and as fast as you try to scramble out you feel that you have slipped back in again! You don't feel like getting out of bed in the morning, you just feel like pulling the covers over your head and never coming out again! You feel absolutely exhausted, shattered and you don't fully understand what is wrong with you! You have difficulty functioning, you have lost interest in most things, you don't feel motivated, your concentration is impaired, you feel anxious and down and life's pleasures seem to be passing you by!

In addition, you feel that nobody fully understands you, what you are going through and how seriously debilitating it all is! You may have withdrawn from people and don't even feel like answering the telephone, however, isolation only compounds the condition!

You may even feel embarrassed that you are suffering from a condition that falls into the category of 'Mental Health', you may think to yourself that Mental Health issues only happen to 'other people', you might work very hard at trying to disguise your condition and this in itself can add to the exhaustion and despondency.
You may be suffering so badly that you think that you don't want to carry on anymore, but please bear this in mind, 'Don't make the most important decision of your entire life, when you are not in the right state of mind to do so'.

People have been suffering from and recovering from episodes of mental distress since mankind began and they will continue to do so in the future! We are all human, therefore, we are not perfect and consequently we are all fallible.

WHERE DO YOU START TO RECOVER? Well, acceptance is key! Accept that you have a problem/condition and as with all problems there is usually a solution.

Accept that you may need some help to become well again! To rediscover the old you, especially the parts of the old you that will help you to recover, you may also need to disregard certain aspects that are unhelpful to you.

You feel stuck. In a rut. However, you are now ready to do the work and to make the changes that are necessary to get yourself better, ultimately it is only you who can get yourself better! You may need help, advice, guidance and support along the way but in the end it will be you who gets you better! Please don't underestimate the power of self-help; along with acceptance this is the other key that unlocks the door to recovery.

YOU CAN DO IT AND YOU WILL DO IT! I am not saying that it is going to be easy; in fact it will be tough!

You will need hope, courage, strength, humility, tenacity, perseverance and determination along your journey, however, all journeys have a destination whatever the distance and I assure you that you will eventually get to where you want to be!

So, to summarise:

- You will need to apply acceptance with regards to your own condition
- If you need help you will need to ask for it without being too proud
- You will need to believe in self-help techniques
- You will need hope and courage
- And most importantly, you must value yourself

In addition, you must recognise that you can change and that consequently things will improve for you and you will then be on the road to 'RECOVERY'.

It's absolutely fine to have a past, but try to not let your past affect your future too much!

I wish you all good luck on your journeys.

Take one day at a time!
Keep on keeping on!

'NEW BEGINNINGS – WHAT MAY AT FIRST APPEAR TO BE AN ENDING IS OFTEN A NEW BEGINNING'

Anonymous

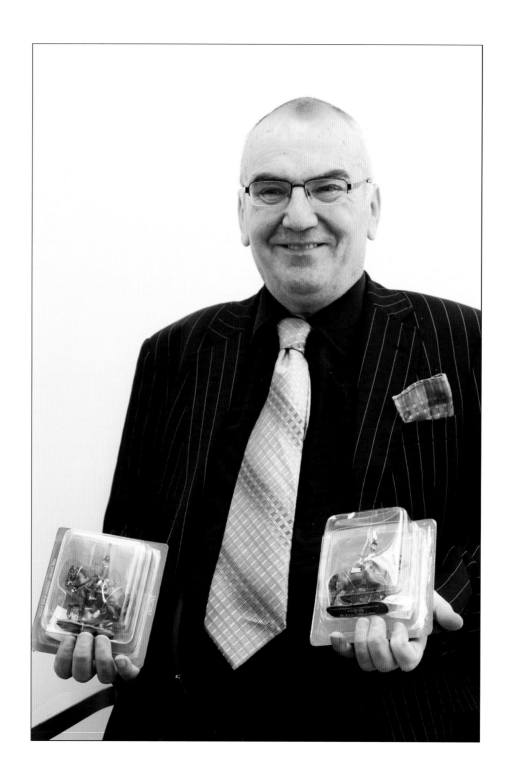

Discovering My Way of Learning

My interest in collecting replicas stems from my father being in the army and spending my childhood searching the secondhand shops for models. I grew up in the 1950's, an era that was dominated by all manner of war films. It was also a time when Britain was starting to lose hold over its empire.

I was fascinated by any soldiers I could find. Some were like new, others had their arms or legs missing, as if they had been chewed off by a young child. There are so many different types that I don't think I'll ever have anywhere near all of them. I really like the variety of regiments and the amazing uniforms.

My knowledge of history has developed through studying the different soldiers from a whole range of campaigns. And not just from a British perspective. For example, how the American Civil War where many nationalities and cultures had representatives fighting on both sides of the conflict. Another fact I learned was that there was a Greek Civil War. I would imagine very few people know that.

My collection numbers well over 200 now. Some are away being mended having lost arms, legs or weapons. They are being 'treated for their injuries'!

I know my fascination isn't shared by everyone. My sister is often criticising the number of soldiers I have and says 'can't you get rid of some of them?'.

But my hobby has led to learning and you can never learn enough.

Declan Hanifan

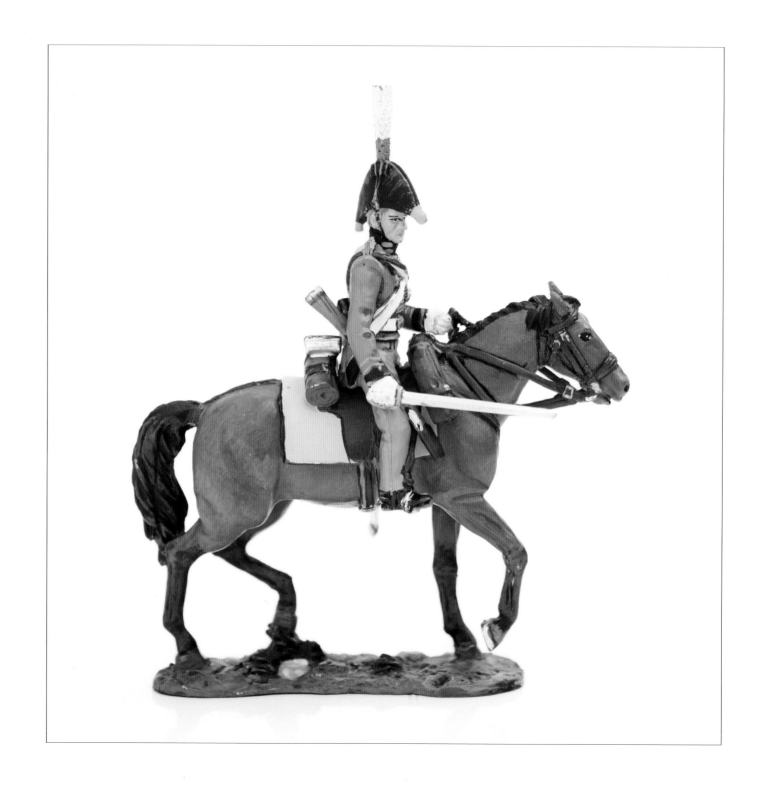

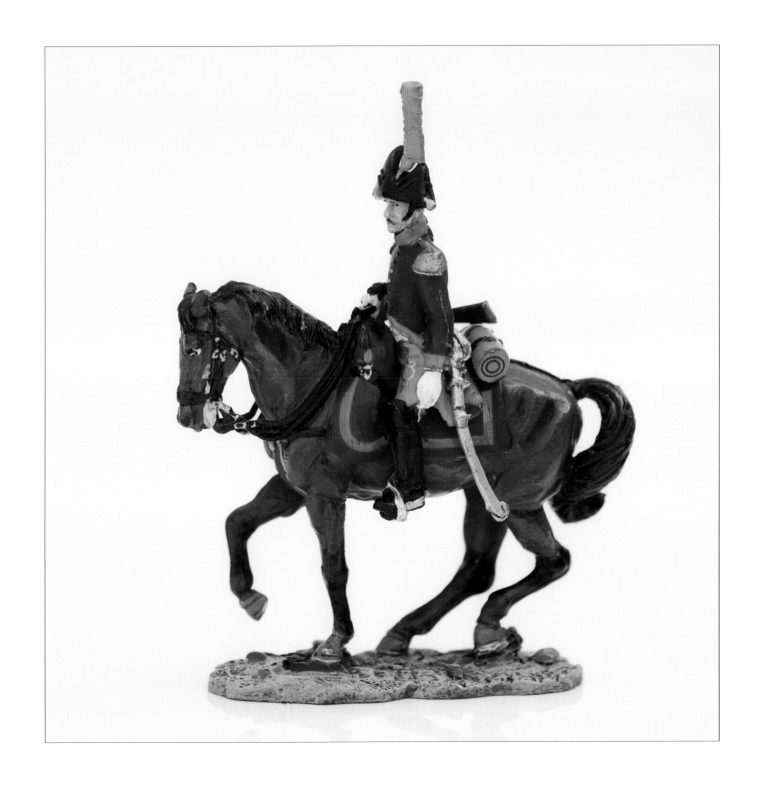

Recovery Is. . . becoming involved

I would like to emphasise my own personal journey towards recovery. I was first diagnosed with a serious mental illness in 1977, some 33 years ago and my mental health has been a prime facet of most of the rest of my life since then. Like many friends with mental health issues, I have always 'recovered' in the sense that following discharge (and I have been incarcerated in psychiatric institutions some 9 times now) I have attempted to pick up the threads of life in the world and have been lucky enough to have professional qualifications and find a route back to work.

Recovery in that sense is nothing new to me but the term has recently been recast as the 'recovery model' which ideally supports each client's potential for recovery. The term has gained particular credence following deinstitutionalisation and the emphasis on community treatment. Support Time and Recovery workers have been appointed throughout the mental health services and it is seen as an idea 'whose time has come'.

I propose therefore to briefly outline my own journey to recovery following my last hospitalisation in 2003. Following twenty years of marriage which broke down in 2000 and difficulties encountered at work I was admitted on three occasions between the years 2000 and 2003. My first instinct was to do what I had always done – seek to return to work and I did this for some time following discharge. But increasingly I found formal paid employment to be stressful and not for me any longer. I decided to plough a new furrow into which I could divert my new found energies.

I 'became involved' in the service user movement locally. I was elected Chair of the HUBB advocacy organisation. This addressed the following areas of my recovery. Hope – a willingness to persevere and pursue a new identity. Self – a regaining of a durable sense of self including self-esteem and social belonging. Empowerment and self determination - having confidence in decision making and feeling in control. Coping strategy – self-management of my time and energies whilst having a structure to my life. Meaning - developing a sense of one's meaning and purpose in life.

Subsequently, I have expanded on this role by being elected a public governor of the North East London NHS Trust and a trustee of Havering MIND. Some weeks my diary seems quite full and I am 'not working'! I honestly feel that these activities have supported my mental health in the last few years sufficiently to keep me away from requiring any further hospital treatment. I do not put forward voluntary work as a universal panacea – the essence of the recovery approach is that it should suit the client and empower the disempowered in whatever ways are appropriate and acceptable. Finally, it needs to be stated that the recovery narrative may not suit every client and we have to strive against the thinking which is sometimes advanced that recovery ultimately implies 'getting back to work' with the implied threats of removal of benefit and other necessary support for vulnerable individuals.

Neil Wood

The Jim Jam Walk

It was a challenging start, walking along a pebbled beach, watching green t-shirts stream ahead of us. The sky was blue and the sun still hot as 3 of us began the 9 miles sponsored walk from Cooden Beach to Eastbourne to raise money for the local St Wilfred's hospice. None of us had walked anything like that distance for at least 30 years!

At Norman's Bay there were no green t-shirts in sight. That's when we started to lose heart. Our feet were aching; our light-weight bags straining our shoulders. Healthy apples and nuts & raisins didn't hit the spot; in fact they were firmly rejected as we contemplated ways of jumping ship.

Step by blistered step we kept moving forwards, and e-v-e-n-t-u-a-l-l-y we were greeted in Pevensey by a steward, guiding us into the pub – the rest-stop. 'Only drinks for the walkers' one customer cried. What a joy to queue for the ladies' toilet and have the chance to chat to other human walkers and compare struggles and cramps.

Off again, determined, refreshed, encouraged…but, soon enough, the straight long road that lead to Sovereign Harbour sapped our strength. Weak smiles met the enthusiastic hoots and encouragements shouted by Sunday drivers. We wove through the Harbour complex, a little uncertain, directed by fresh looking police cadets. The sun was setting as we called for re-enforcements.

John, our Recovery worker, walked out from Eastbourne to meet us. Immediately we split into 2 possies: the 'striders' and the 'strollers'. Encouragement at regular intervals along the sea front kept us going. As we passed the pier the stewards and the organisers swept us up from behind and gathered in their collective embrace, we were cajoled the last few 100 metres to the Big Sleep Hotel.

At 10.30pm, our exhausted bodies made their way up the carpeted stairs of the hotel, expectant of (thick steaming) Hot Chocolate and (those big American) cookies. The digestives had run out and the hot chocolate was from a machine but our evening was immediately worthwhile as 'Jack' from Eastenders put his arms around our shoulders and grinned with us at the camera.

It only (!) took us 3 ½ hours but we're still enjoying the memories and goodwill; and we've raised nearly £150 pounds for the hospice, and that's just 3 of the 465 participants.

By Cynthia and Maggie
Sussex Oakleaf's

Story of Hope and Recovery

I hadn't been going out for about 9 months when a big change happened in my life that brought me confidence. I felt worthwhile and felt the energy of bouncing ideas and watching them snowball nicely.

I had been shown how to colourfully paint cigarette lighters with nail varnish and was sitting in the park one day painting a cigarette lighter when an Irish lady started speaking to me, telling me that she had been attacked in the park. Instead of letting this get me down I decided to brighten up the park and make it a safer place by encouraging people to enjoy it and use it. I began to paint the bench and then the railings. I painted colours and twirls. I painted white and pink and blue in dark places to brighten them up.

People encouraged me. I painted when it was dark to encourage the kids to be there. I suggested building a tea shed/shelter to create a space for people to meet up and get to know each other. I met so many people, especially the Mums and Dads. I also had an idea of a table for old clothes so people could exchange them for free. One fella I met had a friend inside. He asked 'Can I paint my friend's name on a tree?' So that his friend would know that he had been thought about when he was inside.

I stayed in the park from morning to night. A girl told me she felt safe when I was in the park. People asked if I wanted to be a park keeper. I didn't want to do that as that would mean being an authority figure and I didn't want to be that. Others suggested that I paint houses for a job -but I didn't want to do it as a job. I wanted to build and paint sheds different colours for kids to play in. I wanted to make a wishing well.

For all I did and gave I got more back. Like one night a fox, which had been getting used to me, came right up to me and sniffed my feet. When I told people about this they said I would be able to tame the fox to walk around with me - I am good with animals.

Contributed by Andrew Law of 'Tulip'
on behalf of a service user who
wishes to remain anonymous

Recovery Is...

The Great Outdoors

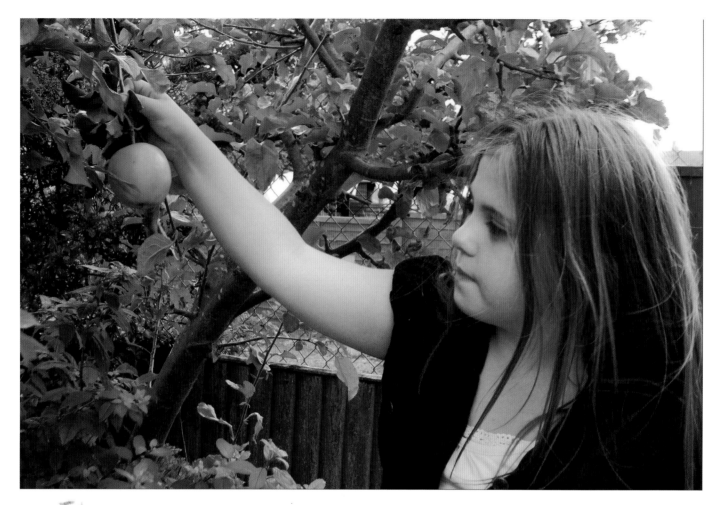

I'm showing my Granddaughter how much fun can be had in the Garden and a sense of achievment when plants and food grow. Here she is picking an apple in her great Grandmother myra's Garden. Bayleigh is the apple of my eye.

Denise Miller

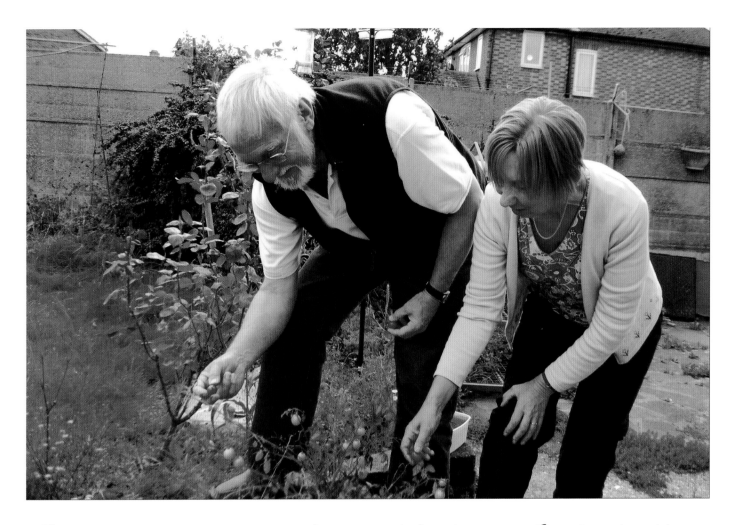

This is a very nice couple I met last year. Gordon is the chairman of the Friends of Havering Conservation Team and Joan, his wife, is the Secretary.

Here they are picking ripe tomotoes in their garden.

Denise Miller

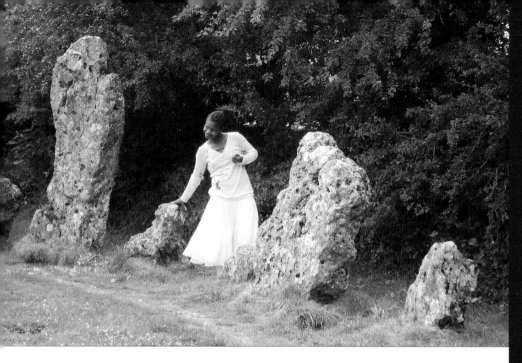

Archaeology and Rock

From 'Eight foundation stones of this gangrel recovery'

Jeremy Voaden

Fougous, chambered cairns, circles of stone. Built by our intelligent and creative ancestors, whose wondrous awareness embraced astronomy, ecology, magnetism and hard work . I have found over many years, that the dreams I have sleeping inside burial chambers vary depending upon which part I am lying in.

Curled inside the side-chambers beneath huge sky-slabs in West Kennett, lying full stretch along the cervical representation in stone of Belas Knapp, spotting shooting stars atop Wayland Smithy.

There is something inside me that speaks to me and says that I have always been here in this place and that I belong here. The sense of belonging is so comforting to me. The awareness of the place and where it stands in the wider landscape. It gives me a feeling of protection (or resilience) against the wear and tear. I carry the protection away with me but can revisit, celebrate, sleep and re-charge at any time.

For just over thirty years I have spent solstices at the Rollright Stones, most recently as a member of the Cotswold Order of Druids. Ceremony. Burial. Re-birth. These places are 'nests' for me.

Sometimes we recite:
"Ancestors, grant us your protection,
And in Protection, Strength,
And in Strength, Understanding,
And in Understanding, Knowledge,
And in Knowledge, the Knowledge of Justice...."

Sometimes, just silence.

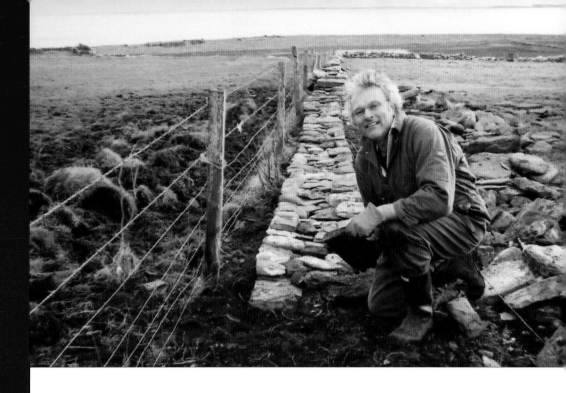

Walking. Wander across the wolds, or parts of Orkney, I see a wall and think "I built that" or, more usually, re-built or repaired that. It feels good.

One key element of a dry stone wall is the 'fill', the small or tiny chippings that I place into the spaces between the larger stones at the heart of the wall. It is entirely possible to build a wall without 'fill'. Such walls look good from the outside, the weakness cannot be seen. They tumble and part much more readily in the ice, snow or freeze-thaw snow and when livestock scratch and itch against the stone.

Building walls is my practical and emotional 'fill'.

Dry-stone walling

From 'Eight foundation stones of this gangrel recovery'

Jeremy Voaden

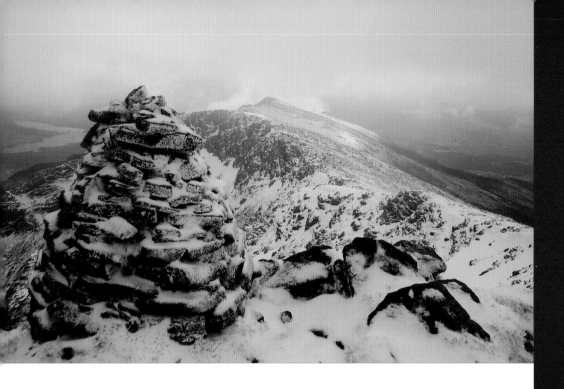

Walking in the Scottish hills

From 'Eight foundation stones of this gangrel recovery'

Jeremy Voaden

There is no-one else here.

On my own but not alone.

Compass, map, line of ridge,
incision of water.

Wander.

Days open up ahead of footfall.

Freedom.

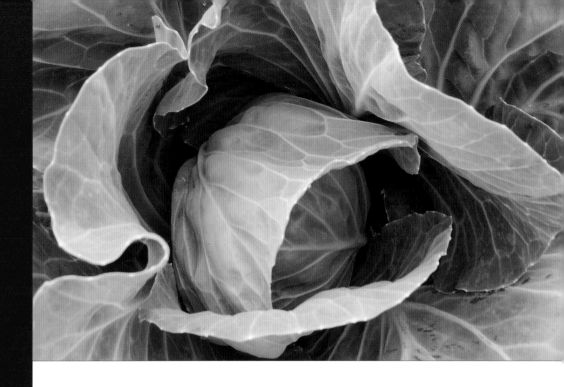

Scratch the leaves of a walnut tree and inhale the scent of the oil.

Smear over-ripe raspberries on my lips and lick it off.

Cook a rhubarb and blackcurrant crumble and serve it to my children for tea, mid-winter, with custard.

Allotment

From 'Eight foundation stones of this gangrel recovery'

Jeremy Voaden

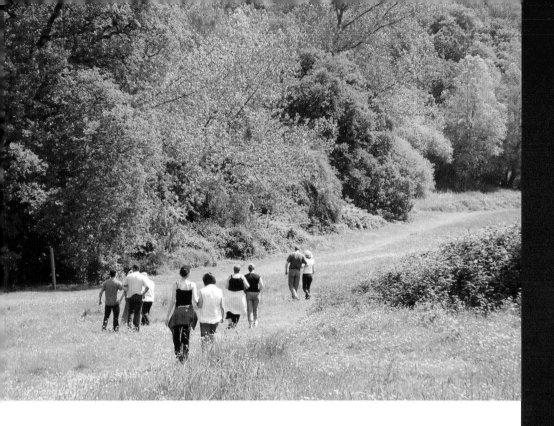

FREE TIME

I watch the tree branches
swaying in the breeze

When my emotions churn up
then freeze

Learn how to stand
strong and grounded

Tell my brain I will not be hounded

Relax my jaw, unclench my fingers

Believe in myself

And only the soft breeze lingers

*Contributed by a member of the
Ecotherapy Group*

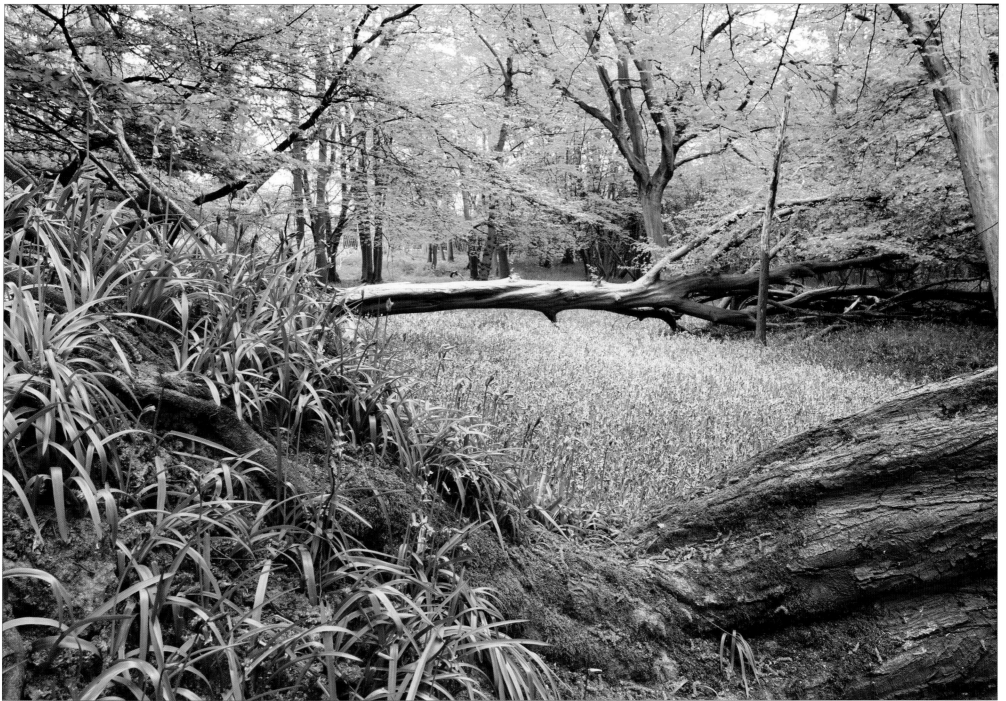

83

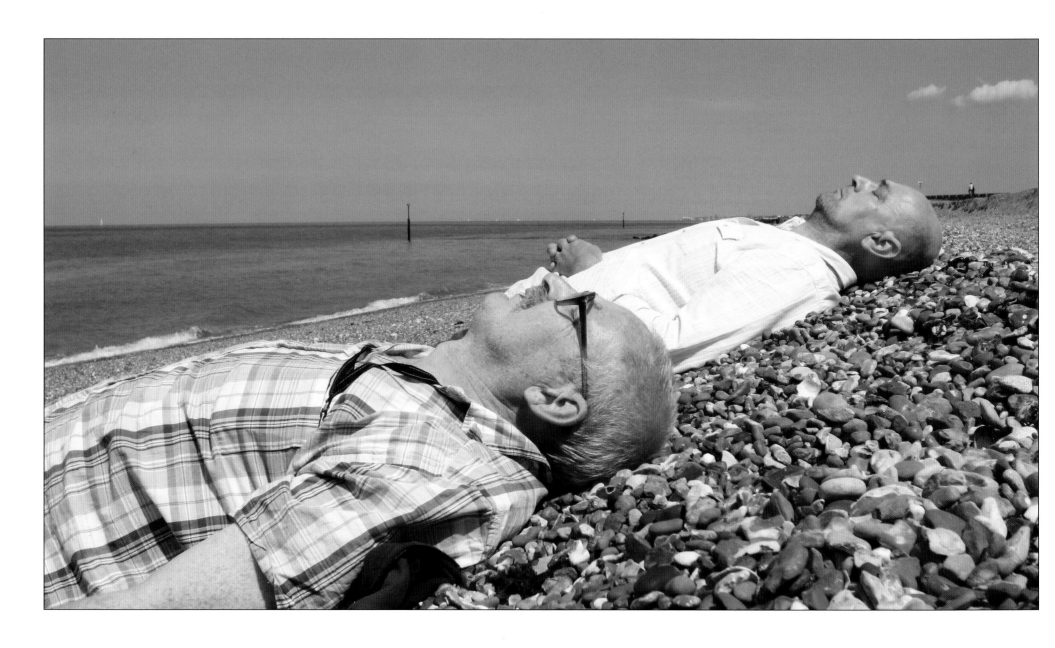

Service User Comments on Ecotherapy

GN

'It is relaxing and gives you space to collect your thoughts. It is something I look forward to, much better than staying indoors.'

SS

'Ecotherapy has helped ease my depression. Even if I didn't feel low I would still come on these walks. It is so relaxing and stepping back from the hustle and bustle of a town, appreciating woodland, is something everyone should do.'

AM - woman in late 30's

'Now I have started doing conservation work on the Fit n' Green Project and I'm getting a lot out of that. I like to be involved and I'm not satisfied with just going round the shops. You know the trees are going to be there for children in the future so I like to do some thing to protect Nature. Purpose is important, to be able to look forward to a day and do something positive. The conservation work means you are not so self absorbed, it takes you out of yourself, it takes your mind off yourself and then you get a chain reaction, you start something going and you become normal again.

Nature does not ask anything of you. I remember when I was feeling low going out on my walks in Bedfords Park and watching squirrels chasing each other or birds fighting and smiling to myself, it is a different world. At the time of my breakdown I didn't like to be with people but I could be at one with Nature. It is alive... it has been a gradual journey from childhood really and I feel better in myself. Nature is something deeper, I think you know what I mean, it feeds the soul.'

Conversations with Ecotherapy Group Members

B's Story

I like the exercise, getting oxygen into you and being outdoors in the countryside. I like to be outdoors but I don't feel safe on my own as a woman, so I don't go out. I'm not isolated at home but it is good to meet other people here, people with similar interests. When you are working you have company here, not like housework when you are on your own. I have learnt about myself, the main thing is motivation. I didn't see myself as competitive but when I see others working I want to work as well and when I work in the garden at home I give up easily when I've had enough. Others fire you on to do more just by being with them, not what anyone says.

'F' said last week that he nearly gave up but he said it got him out of the four walls at home in the day and he can see his girlfriend in the evenings. He liked doing something useful as well.

I have also learnt about the flora and fauna. I thought to myself, I've got to this age (I'm 60 now) and I don't know the different types of common trees and birds. When I usually go for a walk I don't learn about the birds. We need a handout or notes or something so I can look at it again and remember the trees, berries, leaves, and birds we have seen. Sue liked taking pictures of the mushrooms didn't she and sending the pictures to her friends.

As an out-patient I don't meet up with other patients, not that I always want to be with other patients or service users as we are called now. I don't like going out to Romford at night with all the crime and muggings so I don't join in and meet other patients much. When I come out to 'Fit 'n' Green' in the countryside my problems go, I don't get anxious. I don't think of anything else. I say to myself, there is nothing wrong with me in the countryside. I get a booster of confidence doing this. I achieve new things, I've learnt how to use the tools and do the job.

A relative says this project has transformed me. It's had an effect on me doing work at home, I feel more motivated to do things and get on with it because I know I have less time if I'm coming out to Thames Chase. I see housework in a different light – I make light work of it if I'm going out, I do things quicker. Motivation is very important, this fires me up. I set my sights on things now. I keep up to date.

I think you have to get people on this just at the right time. When I came out of hospital it took a little while to get into the swing of things, back into a routine. Then the Occupational Therapist and CPN recommended me to 'Fit 'n' Green' to help me get back into more of a routine. The CPN and O/T work hand in hand with Thames Chase, you are not left on your own, they work in partnership.

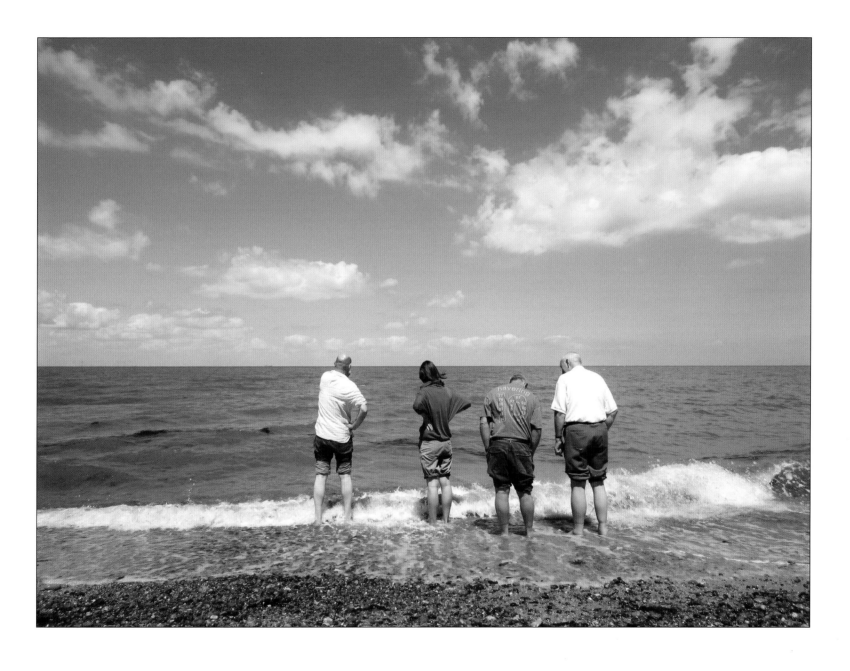

'I feel happier. It lifts my spirits being out. It's like a holiday to me.'

Recovery Is...

Animals

Recovery is...

I've spent the last seven years talking about recovery and training others in what it means to me but not until I was asked to comment as part of this project, have I really considered what recovery is.

It is more than merely a word. It represents something different to every individual and is more of an approach, ethos or way of living. It is not a model.

Recovery is founded on hope. Not the 'hope-I-win-the-lottery' kind of hope but the belief that life can and will be better. Stories of recovery are vital to spreading the message that life can be lived alongside symptoms of mental distress and can inspire others to explore their own journey. Maybe recovery is better described as 'discovery' or 're-discovery' as we learn new ways of living that go beyond coping, managing or surviving. For me recovery is about thriving and moving towards my goals and dreams for a meaningful and personally fulfilling life. I am aware that I may experience setbacks and may even face future hospital admissions, but I will endeavour to make the most of the opportunities I have been given.

I am fortunate to live in a beautiful part of the world and I feel closest to recovery when I am walking my precious dog, Ella, in the woods near my home. A word that isn't often mentioned in recovery and one that I confess to not using much in my talks, is love. When I first saw the title of this project I immediately recalled the 'Love is....' cartoons that were very popular when I was growing up. I'm convinced that knowing you are loved and being able to express love for others is an important part of recovery. Love comes in many forms, be it love for a partner, a parent, a child, a pet or God. A common thread through many recovery stories is faith and how people have made sense of their experiences with a strong belief in God or accepting that there is a Higher Power.

I mentioned earlier the word 'journey' and how many people talk of their recovery in terms of a journey. For me a journey conjures up thoughts of holidays or visiting relatives in far flung places. I personally think my journey is more accurately described as a 'quest.' That's not to say I'm a Frodo Baggins kind of character but a quest generates thoughts of adventure, hurdles to overcome, raging rivers to cross and mountains to climb. Also, from quest we derive the word question and throughout my life I have constantly been asking questions of myself. I have never claimed to hear 'voices' but these questions like 'Why am I here?', 'What am I doing?' and 'Where am I going?' have never been far from my thoughts.

As well as hope, recovery is about choice, acceptance and responsibility. I choose how I react to my diagnosis and how I engage with people who look after me when I am unwell. In recent years I have accepted that these people have my best interests at heart and ultimately want what I want: to get back on with living my life. It took a long time to reach this acceptance as I was trained as a soldier and spent years not trusting my care providers which led to many instances of absconding and reacting angrily to staff. It wasn't until a relapse led to a serious crime that I realised my attitude had to change. It was whilst in secure services in 2004 that I first heard about recovery and made a conscious decision to work alongside and in partnership with staff. Just a few years after leaving that hospital I was driving myself back through the gates as a recovery trainer. This was a personal moment of triumph and I was gradually taking on the responsibility of being a self-employed recovery speaker and trainer, firmly believing that I could make a good living using my hard-won experience to help others. Six years later I am still self-employed and loving the work I do despite having been hospitalised three times in the past four years. I now view relapses as 'research' and although I appreciate the strain these put on my marriage, each time I emerge stronger and wiser.

So there it is, a little slice of what recovery is to me and the photos are of Ella and one taken of me speaking at a recovery conference in Dublin.

James Wooldridge

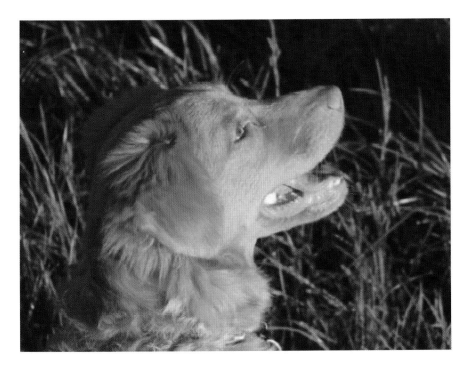 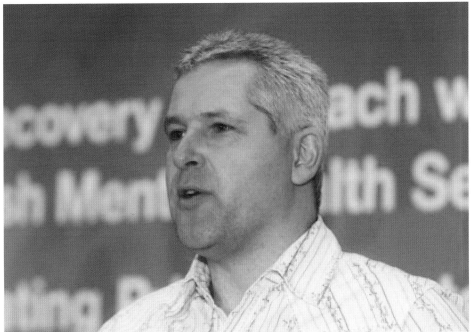

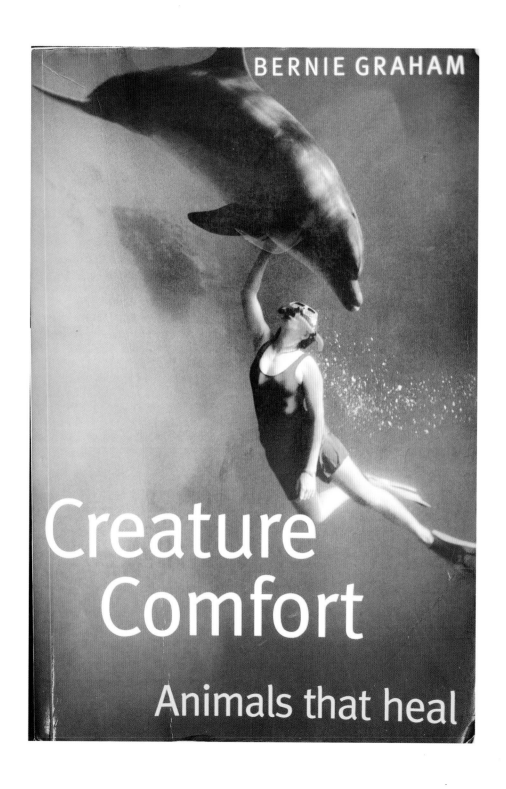

BERNIE GRAHAM

Creature Comfort

Animals that heal

There is nothing quite like the old style British mental hospital. The often tranquil rural settings cannot compensate for the intimidating red brick Victorian institutional architecture. Even though I've visited many of my clients in such places over the last decade who have found themselves both voluntary and involuntary recipients of care on draughty wards, my feelings of unease on entering these surroundings remain undiminished. However, on this occasion I was a little less apprehensive. This was primarily due to the presence of Max, a six month old black Labrador puppy, who had placed his head inches from mine as he eagerly viewed the outside world through the front window of the Volvo. His surprisingly pleasant breath had been caressing my right cheek for most of the thirty minute journey to Napsbury Hospital on the outskirts of north-west London. He had also treated me to the occasional ear licking, which I would like to report as a supportive response to my increasing anxiety but this would be deceitful, since Max was most undiscriminating in what he licked. In fact as we drove through the hospital gates I suddenly remembered the last part of his own anatomy he had licked before me.

Max's 'owner' Julia McAvoy and I were visiting Liam, a resident of the mental health housing project we were both involved in. He had been in hospital for several weeks suffering from a quite severe bout of depression. Liam was especially fond of Max and had looked after him on several occasions. We had informed him the day before that we were bringing the dog up for a visit and it was clear from his response that he was very excited about seeing him again. It was to be Max's first visit to the hospital and, given his extremely lively nature, we thought it best he didn't enter the wards. The plan was that while Julia visited another client, Liam and I would take him for a walk.

As we progressed further into the hospital grounds following the directions to Larch ward, the grotesquely ornate water tower came into view. This was a particularly intimidating feature of the hospital. It was no more than 150 feet high but it had the presence of a structure twice its size. It's styling appeared an unfortunate hybrid of Gothic and what I can only describe as Babylonian features. It was as though a beacon had been erected, to proclaim to all who entered the hospital, the indisputable dominance of the Victorian institution.

We eventually arrived at the ward. Max was itching to get out and explore this unfamiliar place.

It was initially necessary to keep him on a leash in case other patients and staff were less inclined to make his acquaintance. I stayed with him while Julia went to collect Liam. When she returned there was quite a reunion. Max and Liam were very pleased to see each other. After five to ten minutes of jumping, licks and hugs, Liam and I took Max for a run in the extensive grounds. We headed for a more secluded area so we could take the straining canine off the leash. We chatted in between throwing a stick and playing tug of war with Max. Liam explained that he was feeling a little more positive and was hoping to return to the housing project in the very near future. We also talked about football and the less-than-delightful hospital food. Throughout our conversation Liam rarely took his eyes off Max and smiled more readily than I had seen him do for some time. We spent an hour or so together before returning to the ward to meet Julia.

Max reluctantly got in the car and Liam said his final farewells through the window. Julia and myself said our goodbyes to Liam and commented on how much brighter he seemed. He agreed and repeated his desire to return home as soon as possible.

As we got in the car Liam gave Max a toothy grin. Julia said it was good to see him smile again. He chuckled and informed us that a nurse had also noticed him smiling earlier in the day and he recounted their conversation,

"In all the weeks that you've been on the ward I have never seen you smile first thing in the morning- it's good to see."
"Well today is different" Liam responded.
"Why?" the nurse enquired.
He smiled again, "Well today Max is coming to see me."

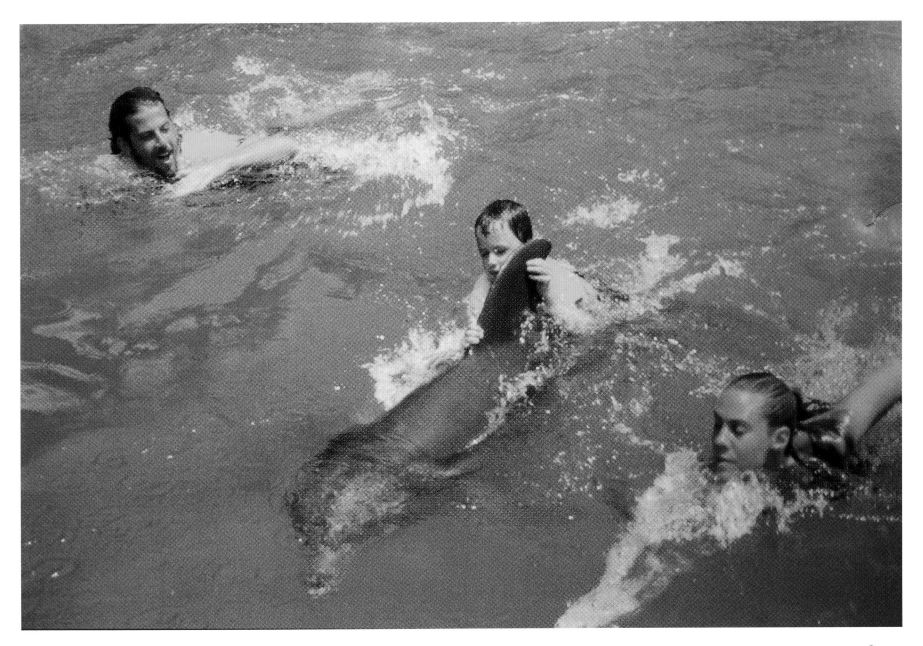

Bernie Graham

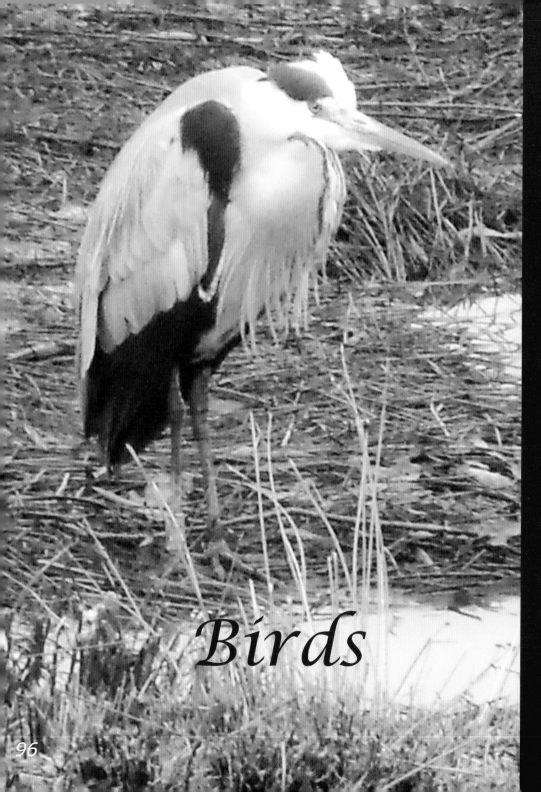

Birds

'Sparkle out into the blue- Not ours any more'

Ted Hughes 'Swifts'

Some Swifts have lived for more than 10 years, but assuming a lifespan of 7 years, then such a bird would have flown more than 1.28 million miles, never landing during its life other than to breed.

Wonder.

The feelings I have thinking on this must be close to happiness. I feel in awe but not afraid, I feel the birds bring me a focus, in time, of seasons, and understanding of connections between things. Each year they return.

Safety, expectation, anticipation.

The joy of the first sight.

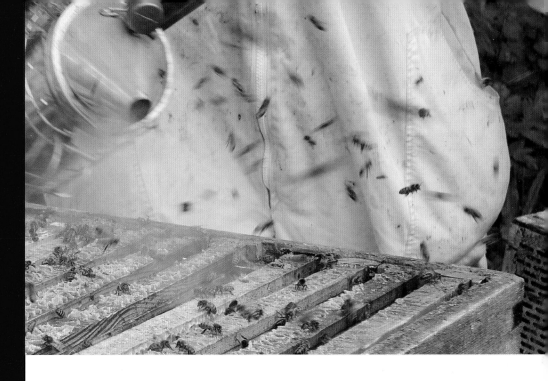

Opening a hive focuses my mind. I have never heard voices working the frames. Rhythm, concentration, observation, pain, delight. Now I find I am beginning to anticipate the temperament of the bees from their smell. The pheremones they are giving off. Knowing there is always more to know and the pleasure of the learning. The putting of it into practice. Testing, making mistakes, caring for them. Bees have been at the centre of my recovering compass for the last decade.

Wonder.

BEES

From 'Eight foundation stones of this gangrel recovery'

Jeremy Voaden

Jeff Walker

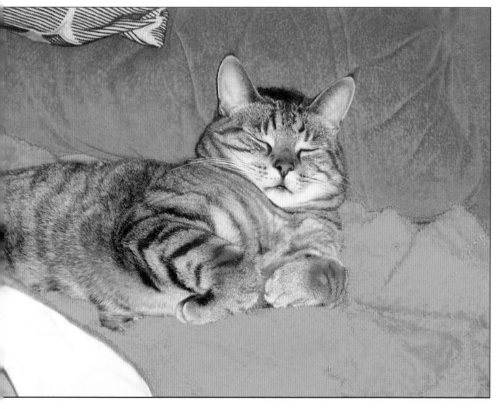

Saffie is the cat on the left. George is the one on the right and currently chewing on my elbow as he sits on some paperwork that I am working on.

I adopted Saffie just after coming out of hospital after an attempt to take my own life. A very good friend of mine took me for lunch and then took me to the Bristol Dogs Home, which also helps lost and abandoned cats. My friend's rationale was that she knew I would not attempt to take my own life again if I had a cat to look after – I would not let the cat be left alone in my house and/or go back to the dogs home.

When I arrived at the cattery, I was somewhat reluctant to choose a cat. I notice one cat jump up as soon as I walked near to her cage, which touched me somewhat, so I said I wanted that cat. My friend, having previously visited the cattery section, knew the cat I was talking about and advised me against adopting her, but to look at some other cats first.

Apparently the cat in question was a bit 'difficult'. She fouled and wet the carpet, did not like children was anti social and very timid. I thought, 'that's the cat for me'. My friend continued to try to have me look at other cats, but I kept on saying I want that one (long before Andy in the wheelchair said it in Little Britain).

Eventually, I did adopt the cat, who I named Saffie.

When she moved in, she spent about three weeks living behind the fridge. I used to sit near the fridge and talk to her, each day I would move her food a little further away from the fridge to encourage her to come out. Eventually she did move out from behind the fridge – she moved under one of the base units in the kitchen. From there she moved behind the sofa. After about six weeks to two months, she finally poked her head from behind the sofa and allowed me to stroke her. From then on, we became inseparable and she was a fantastic cat. She never fouled or wet on the carpet. She remained timid, but not with me. She would come and sleep on my chest, especially when I was depressed or low. Saffie was part of my recovery as she needed me and took me out of my negative space where all I could focus on was my depression.

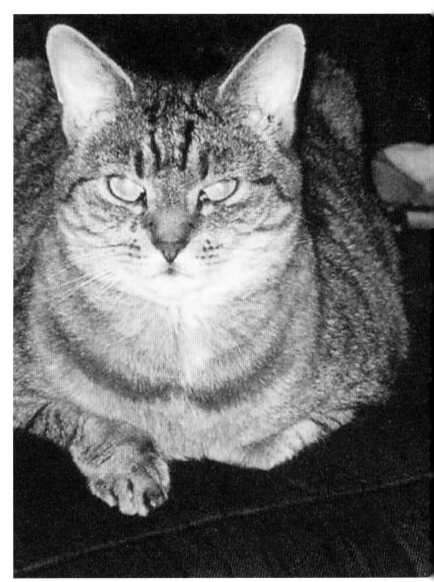

Sadly, Saffie died (peacefully) a couple of years after I adopted her (cancer). I like to think she had a good last few years.

About six months after Saffie died, a friend asked me if I wanted to have another cat. I said no, but went along to the dogs home regardless. I ended up adopting two cats that day – George and Mildred. Mildred eventually left home and moved in with a neighbour. She still pops in occasionally. George is a completely different cat to Saffie – I think I am a different person to when I adopted her or I am in a different place. George is very affectionate and very confident – he loves people and attention.

Jeff Walker

I Painted a broken terracotta flower pot, upended it to see what would live in it. There has been snailes and Toads because of the moisture and protection from the Sun.

Denise Miller

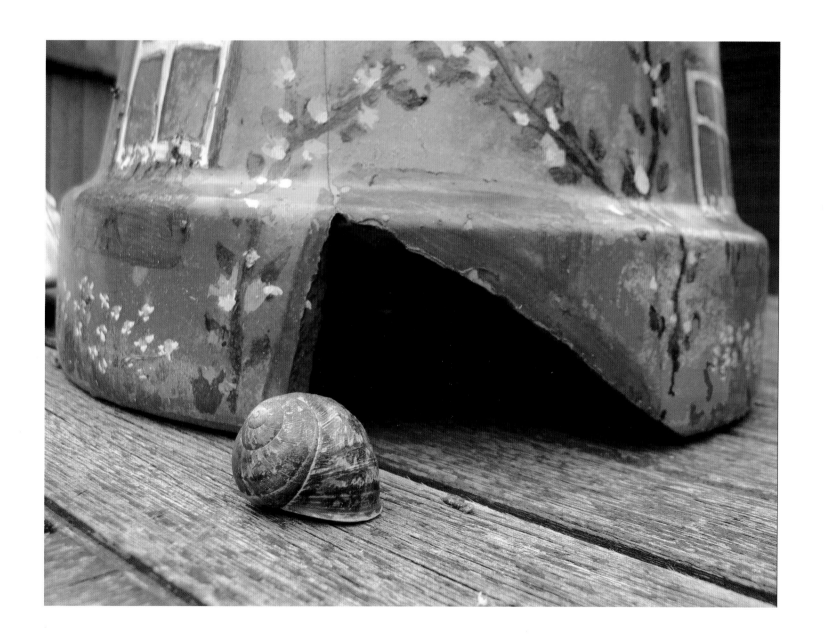

Recovery Is...

Top Tips

The Recovery Route is not easy. It entails taking personal responsibility.

It involves challenging, not just providers of mental health services, or friends and family – but yourself most of all. There are sign-posts on the recovery route – and these all help you to regain balance and control.

There are however, no magic answers to prevent you becoming unwell at some time. Recovery is not about that. It is also not about having to be medication-free, or never using services again.

Recovery is about taking back control of the wheel of your car instead of sitting in the passenger seat – just going along for the ride

I'd like recovery for the 'helping professionals' to be this:

1. Be an ambassador for hope

2. However scared I am that I'm not going to get better, be equally strong in your conviction that I will

3. Understand the various diagnoses fully, and how they can be expressed differently for each individual so you don't get my symptoms confused with 'me'

4. Remember, no one gets 'diplomatic immunity' from mental distress, not even you

5. Be led by me. You would be surprised by what I know about myself

6. Think of someone you love, a daughter, a friend, a mother needing the support from another professional that I need from you. Treat me the same as you would have them treated. After all, I am someone's daughter, friend and mother too

7. Ask about my hopes and dreams and plans, ask about what I have achieved – and hope to achieve

8. Encourage my independence

9. Don't hide behind your job title. If I can't see who you are behind it, then how can I expect you to see who I am behind my 'diagnosis'?

10. Be the best that you can be

Anonymous

Top Ten Tips for Recovery

- Learning to be in the driving seat of your own journey of self discovery

- Learning on your journey it may have ups and downs that we are not always reasonable for but we are in charge of choices we make to life's ups and downs

- To take positive risks that will help us in our endeavor to develop a meaningful life

- To develop a jigsaw without always knowing what the picture will look like

- To take time out for ourselves in pursuit of things we enjoy doing

- To develop coping strategies that feel right for us

- Learning to say no to things that have a negative impact on our emotional wellbeing

- Learning to believe we can work towards the right to have good things in our life

- To work towards being comfortable in our own skin

- It is ok to make mistakes as this is part of life's rich tapestry!

Lynn Burling

Five Simple Tools

Connect:

Connect with the people around you. With family, friends, colleagues and neighbours. At home, work, school or in your local community. Think of these as the corner of your life and invest time in developing them. Building these connections will support and enrich you every day.

Be active:

Go for a walk or a run. Step outside. Cycle. Play a game. Garden. Dance. Exercising makes you feel good. Most importantly, discover a physical activity you enjoy and one that suits your level of mobility and fitness.

Take notice:

Be curious. Catch sight of the beautiful. Remark on the usual. Notice the changing seasons. Savour the moment, whether you are walking to work, eating lunch or talking to friends. Be aware of the world around you and what you are feeling. Reflecting on your experiences will help you appreciate what matters to you.

Keep learning;

Try something new. Rediscover an old interest. Sign up for that course. Take on a different responsibility at work. Fix a bike. Learn to play an instrument or how to cook your favourite food. Set a challenge you will enjoy achieving. Learning new things will make you more confident as well as being fun.

Give:

Do something nice for a friend, or a stranger. Thank someone. Smile. Volunteer your time. Join a community group. Look out, as well as in. Seeing yourself, and your happiness, linked to the wider community can be incredibly rewarding and creates connections with the people around you.

Jeff Walker

A list of good advice for good mental health

Think the right thoughts, try to think positive thoughts, try not to think negative thoughts. Think about good things, do not think about bad things.

Have something to do, to keep your mind occupied.

Do not take on too many things to do, so you don't get too stressed.

Have enough rest. Have the right balance of rest and activity.

Have a hobby or leisure activity to help you to relax.

Be aware of your own emotions. Learn to express your strong emotions in a way that is acceptable to other people. Do not keep emotions bottled up inside you.

Listen to music, music can be a way of expressing emotions.

Live a good life. Avoid doing things that are wrong, to avoid guilt feelings, which can make you feel depressed.

Have a social life, get out and meet people, do not be reclusive.

Face up to life's problems, face up to reality, do not ignore problems.

Accept that some problems are a part of everyday life.

Find ways of dealing with problems, as a way of improving how you deal with life.

Talk to other people about ways of dealing with problems.

If a situation becomes too difficult to deal with, get away from it if you need to - "I can't take any more of this."

Have some goals in life, something to aim for, to keep you going.

Aim for the right kind of things in life.

We all need someone to tell us we are 'all right', that we are a 'good person'.

Tell yourself you are OK, to improve your own self esteem.

Tell other people that they are 'all right', tell them they are OK.

Hazel & John Radford

Thou

Thou shalt not cling,
Thou shalt not clutch.
Depend on others over much.
Thou shalt not meddle or condemn.
The souls of others leave to them.
Thou shalt not harbour bootless care.
Thou shalt not give but freely share.
No sap of life do thou destroy.
All things by faith thou shalt enjoy.
Don't lean on those thou holdest dear.
Above all else THOU SHALT NOT FEAR.

Anonymous

Recovery Is...

About You!

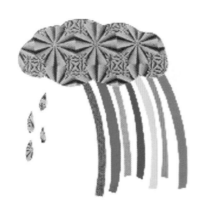

In the hour of adversity be not without hope
For crystal rain falls from black clouds

Autumn Hardy

We hope you will have been inspired by the many different ways our contributors have approached their own recovery journeys. What is important to their recovery, maintaining their wellbeing and how it can be expressed in many forms.

These last pages are about YOU! They have been left free for you to add your own work. Anything, in any way, that will help you on your own recovery journey.

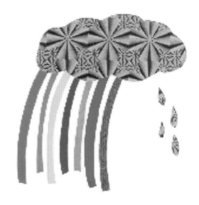

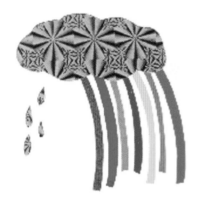

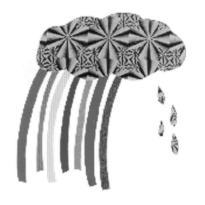

And now you have added your work, pick up this book now and again to remind yourself of what you and others have achieved.

It may be the start of you creating your own 'Recovery Is...' Book!

Acknowledgements

HUBB's first insights into recovery began with James Wooldridge in 2006 who helped us to deliver our first Recovery Seminars – thank you James for setting us on the path and sharing your journey.

Thank you to the HUBB Recovery Team over the past five years:

    Anne Myatt – for the concept of the book
    Anita Coplestone – for organising the original recovery groups
    Lynn Burling – someone whose path on her journey to recovery has proved to be an inspiration to all who meet her
    Suzan Arisoy – whose poems still inspire and who we all miss very much
    Rob Thomas – without whose skills this book would not have become a reality

Thank you to all the contributors to the book and those who have shared their experiences with us.

Metloc Printers Limited of Romford for their publishing expertise.

Huge thanks to the National Lottery – Awards for All whose first grant in 2006 enabled HUBB to facilitate the original Recovery seminars. This book has been generously funded by a second grant from Awards for All.

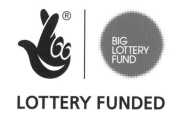

LOTTERY FUNDED